20p

Steve

Science Studies Unit
Univ. of Edinburgh
Feb. 1999

A HISTORY OF THE GENERAL NURSING COUNCIL FOR ENGLAND AND WALES
1919–1969

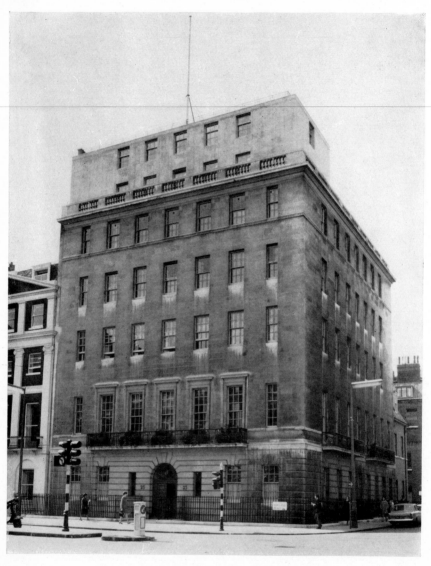

23, Portland Place, London W.1.

A HISTORY OF THE GENERAL NURSING COUNCIL FOR ENGLAND AND WALES 1919 – 1969

by

EVE R. D. BENDALL
S.R.N., R.S.C.N., R.N.T.

and

ELIZABETH RAYBOULD
S.R.N., R.N.T.

Eighteen Illustrations

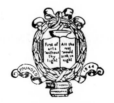

LONDON
H. K. LEWIS & CO LTD
1969

First published 1969

©

H. K. LEWIS & CO LTD

1969

By the same Authors

A GUIDE TO
MEDICAL AND SURGICAL NURSING

232 pages, Demy 8vo. 44 illustrations
£1 5s. net (£1 in limp covers)

BASIC NURSING

134 pages, Demy 8vo. 48 illustrations
Second Edition £1 5s. net (£1 in limp covers)

Standard Book No. 7186 0091 6

PRINTED IN GREAT BRITAIN
BY HAZELL WATSON AND VINEY LTD., AYLESBURY, BUCKS

"On the one hand, the friend who is familiar with every fact of the story may think that some point has not been set forth with that fullness which he wishes and knows it to deserve; on the other, he who is a stranger to the matter may be led to suspect exaggeration if he hears anything above his nature."   PERICLES

PREFACE

It seems, to the authors, that the occasion of the jubilee of the General Nursing Council for England and Wales is a suitable time for the publication of an account of its first 50 years. Although "history of nursing" is listed as one of the subjects in the Council's syllabuses of training for nurses, it is remarkable how little is known or taught of the events recorded in this book. In 1919 there was no statutory training and no national qualification; in 1969 there will be over 500,000 names entered in the Council's Register and Roll and some 70,000 nurses in training.

It was difficult to know where to start, but preliminary investigations convinced us that the fight for registration, which preceded the 1919 Nurses Act, so influenced future events that it had to be included—and this took us back to the 1870s.

It has also been difficult to know what to include and what to leave out, since much of the Council's work is incredibly detailed; we therefore decided that each recurring event would only be described in detail the first time it happened—for example, over the years, there have been many Boards of Examiners appointed, but only the names of those who served on the first one have been given.

We are grateful to the General Nursing Council for their interest in this publication and for making all the records freely available to us; however, the book has been written by us as individuals, and inevitably our viewpoints and ideas have influenced the selection and presentation of material.

Many people have helped us in different ways and we would like to acknowledge our gratitude to the following:

the Boards of Governors of the Charing Cross Group of Hospitals and of the Hospital for Sick Children, Gt. Ormond Street, for special leave in December 1967;

Miss Peggy Nuttall, Editor, the *Nursing Times,* for her wise and constructive criticism of the manuscript;

many of the officers and staff of the General Nursing Council, including the Registrar, the heads of departments, the reception/telephonists, and especially Miss Gibbard and Miss Welch who have never failed to find the information we required, or to check repeated lists of facts;

Dr. A. Walk, a long-standing member of Council and of the Royal Medico-Psychological Association, for his help and interest in the sections relating to mental nurse training;

Miss M. Morrison, Registrar, the Joint Nursing and Midwives Council for N. Ireland, Walter Pyke-Lees, Registrar, the General Medical Council, and David Hindley-Smith, Registrar, the General Dental Council for their prompt, willing and detailed response to requests for comparative facts;

and officials of the Royal British Nurses' Association for the answers to several letters.

Many individuals have written to us, and mention must be made of the following:

Miss H. Dey, C.B.E., ex-Matron of St. Bartholomew's Hospital and Miss J. M. Loveridge, while Matron of St. Bartholomew's Hospital;

David B. B. Fenwick, for sending us a photograph of his grandmother, and giving permission for its publication;

Dorothy E. Furbank, née Sullings, assistant to the accountant at the G.N.C. 1922–5, for the photograph of the staff in 1925;

Mrs. M. C. Barber, née Kerr, ex-vice-president of the British College of Nurses for much information, including the account of Mrs. Fenwick's death;

and Miss G. E. Davies, ex-Registrar of the G.N.C.

We would like to thank the typists who deciphered our manuscript, with its many corrections, the staff of the photographic department at Charing Cross Hospital, our friends and colleagues for their patience, encouragement and tolerance of our fascination with past events, and the many who knowingly and unknowingly have helped us to write this book.

To our publishers, H. K. Lewis & Co. Ltd., we offer our gratitude for their unfailing willingness to discuss our ideas and their continuing interest and help.

We acknowledge our debt to Ethel Gordon Fenwick; as registered nurses for her long fight to secure State Registration for nurses; as authors, for the detailed historical records to be found in the *British Journal of Nurses;* and we agree with her grandson that she was a great, if unconventional, woman.

EVE BENDALL

London, 1968.   ELIZABETH RAYBOULD

CONTENTS

CONTENTS

ILLUSTRATIONS

PRELUDE

"It is a long road from the inception of a thing to its realisa-
tion."   MOLIÈRE

THE GENERAL NURSING COUNCIL TODAY

On the fourth Friday of January, March, May, July, September
and November, at 2.30 p.m., any members of the nursing profession or general public can go to 23 Portland Place, London,
W.1 and take their place in the public gallery of the Council
Chamber to listen to the proceedings of the formal meeting of
the General Nursing Council for England and Wales. The
public gallery is small and usually occupied by representatives
of the nursing press, some of the Council's officers, and a few—
half a dozen or so—members of the profession.

The procedure for the meeting is laid down in The Nurses
Rules Approval Instrument 1961, which is obtainable from Her
Majesty's Stationery Office. As with all formal meetings of
large concerns and/or statutory bodies, the actual events may
appear rather dull and difficult to follow, since they consist of
a recital of recommendations forwarded by the various Committees for the approval of Council. Formal committee procedure is followed.

The meeting is opened by the Chairman of Council, at present
(1968) Miss Grace Watts, Matron of the General Infirmary at
Leeds; on her left sits the Registrar, Miss Mary Henry, who acts
as secretary to the Council and beyond her the chief committee
clerk, Miss L. Gibbard. On the Chairman's right is a seat for
the Council's solicitor, who attends when necessary. The various
members, elected and appointed, sit in four rows facing the
Chairman. The vice-Chairman, Miss Rosamond Hone, Principal Tutor of St. Thomas's Hospital, has a specific seat, but all
other members are seated in strict alphabetical order and a seating
plan and name card is placed at each member's position. Once
the meeting is opened, the minutes of the previous meeting are
received, and signed, apologies for absence read, matters arising
from previous minutes dealt with and correspondence read and
noted. At any time it may be decided to take a matter in camera
if approved and the Chairman seeks formal approval for this.

In the last few years, no matter so marked has been challenged by any individual member of Council, although the policy or wisdom of such action has been the subject of discussion both within and outside the Council. The reasons for debating certain matters in private sometimes appear unnecessary to the uninformed observer, but within the Council itself there seem to be two distinct schools of thought. The more conservative element hold that until the Council have decided on a course of action it is unfair to the training schools to hint that changes are afoot, since change can affect all aspects of nurse training. It is probable too that the rumblings of the first General Nursing Council and the upheavals its public arguments caused are still heard by the few. It must be remembered that in the early 1920s, the then Minister of Health had to intervene to restore order and to some, a repetition of this sort of situation must be avoided at all costs. The more radical members believe that the Council's image is in many ways weakened by the impression of unanimous solidarity on all matters which is in fact rare, since argument, debate and difference of opinion are essential in a democratic structure.

The next item on the agenda is the report of the proceedings of each Committee to the Council. Under the Nurses Act, 1957, and The Nurses Rules, 1961, there are three Statutory Committees, i.e. the Finance, Enrolled Nurses and Mental Nurses Committees and four Standing Committees, i.e. the Registration, Education and Examinations, Investigating and Disciplinary Committees. These reports are presented in turn by the appropriate Chairman, for adoption by Council, and since they will have been fully discussed prior to presentation, it is usual for approval to be given at once. It will be obvious that most of the work and much of the power of the Council is in fact delegated to the various Committees and through them to the full-time officers, i.e. the Registrar, Education Officer, Financial Administrator and other departmental heads and their staffs. The only other headings on the agenda are Notices of Motion and Any Other Business. There is rarely anything under these headings, but in fact any member of Council can present a Notice of Motion to the Registrar. This procedure is used when a member or members of Council wish to raise some point not covered in the current agenda or representing a minority view which would otherwise not become known. This was last used when there was some disagreement on the Council's public statement on the Platt Report on basic nurse education.

The announcement of the date of the next meeting concludes the public part of the proceedings and those in the visitors gallery are asked to leave. The meeting rarely takes more than one hour, but it is the culmination of tremendous activity in Committee and in the Council's offices during the preceding two months.

The rules established a register which was open to those who had been trained in the duties of a nurse and had one year on the staff of a hospital or infirmary.

The chief members of the Matrons' Committee resigned and "determined to unite into a powerful body under the guidance, and with the support, of medical men alone"[5]. The leader of this breakaway group was Mrs. E. G. Fenwick.

Mrs. Ethel Fenwick

Mrs. Fenwick, who before her marriage was Ethel Gordon Manson, had trained as a lady-pupil at Nottingham Children's Hospital and a year later at Manchester Royal Infirmary. She then became a ward sister at The London Hospital and at the age of 24, in 1881, was appointed Matron of St. Bartholomew's Hospital. Six years later she married Dr. Bedford Fenwick, and although she then retired from active nursing she was to dominate the nursing scene and nursing politics for the next 60 years.[6] From the start, it was apparent that Mrs. Fenwick was determined that the emerging nursing profession should be led and organised by nurses: she was prepared in her fight, to seek members of the medical profession as allies in her cause, but would not tolerate "interference" by hospital administrators. She was also an ardent feminist and a friend of Mrs. Pankhurst.

Mrs. Fenwick objected to the proposals put forward by Henry Burdett. She thought that a register of the type he suggested would be quite unselective and spoke of it as "a central registry office, similar to that in vogue for domestic servants"[7]. She led the breakaway group to form the British Nurses' Association.

From this time, nurses who desired registration were divided into two distinct camps, and unfortunately this state of affairs was to lead to many bitter disagreements both before and after the 1919 Registration Act. Time, talent, energy and money were to be wasted on details which became so big that on occasions they totally obscured the main issue.

One group of nurses allied themselves with doctors—and the others mainly with hospital administrators. Among the former was Mrs. Fenwick, and among the latter were Mrs. Wardroper, Matron of St. Thomas's Hospital and Miss Eva Luckes, Matron of The London Hospital. According to one source, Miss Luckes' antipathy to Mrs. Fenwick was personal as well as professional:

Chapter 1

THE FIGHT FOR STATE REGISTRATION
OF NURSES

"A new art and a new science has been created since and within the last forty years. And with it a new profession—so they say; we say, calling." FLORENCE NIGHTINGALE

Following the establishment of organised nurse-training, and particularly of the Nightingale Training School in 1860, the concept of a State Register gradually emerged.

In 1858 a Register was started for medical practitioners and soon after this, teachers began demanding similar status, although they did not achieve it until 1899. Nurses were not far behind; the Editorial of the *Nursing Record* stated, "the time has now arrived for the whole question of the Registration of trained nurses to be set forth in a succinct form before the profession and the public". Dr. (later Sir Henry) Acland made the first reference to this in the foreword of a book he edited for Miss Florence Lees in 1874 (Handbook for Ward Sisters). He wrote, "the Medical Act of 1858 allows women to be Registered as Medical Practitioners: it makes no provision for the registration of trained nurses"[1]. At the time Dr. Acland was President of the General Medical Council.

By 1886 there was a definite movement towards the establishment of some sort of register for nurses; the initiative seems to have come from the Hospitals' Association (an organisation of hospital administrators) who set up a committee to study the possibility. In 1887 a meeting was called to discuss this with matrons of leading hospitals who set up a Sectional Committee of the Association. The Committee held meetings and "arrived at the conclusion that no nurse should be registered who had been trained for less than 3 years—and then disagreement arose"[2]. Henry Burdett, spokesman for the Hospitals' Association, thought that one year's training was sufficient, but "the matrons stood firm for quality not quantity in regard to the register"[3]. The Hospitals' Association Council over-rode the Matrons' Committees' decision and in October 1887 issued a notice saying that "the rules for the register of trained nurses had been printed"[4].

I

"it is traditional that Miss Luckes had been in love with Dr. Fenwick. Be that as it may, there was certainly rivalry between the two women"[8].

On the sidelines, distinct from both groups, was the still powerful Miss Florence Nightingale: she was opposed to State Registration in any form. She felt that the time (1886) was not ripe—that perhaps in 40 years the profession might be ready. State Registration was also a contradiction of all she believed training to be: she saw that it would lead to statutory examinations, and said "devotion, gentleness, sympathy, qualities of overwhelming importance in a nurse, could not be ascertained by public examination". She wrote "nursing has to nurse living bodies and spirits. It cannot be tested by public examination, though it may be tested by current supervision"[9]. She also deplored the profession being split into two camps.

THE BRITISH NURSES' ASSOCIATION

On November 21st, 1887 a meeting of the matrons who disagreed with the Hospitals' Association was held at 20 Upper Wimpole Street, London, W.1. It was decided to call a conference of "The Matrons of the chief British Hospitals"[10], and this was held on December 7th. Forty matrons attended, and with Dr. Bedford Fenwick in the chair, the British Nurses' Association was born.

The object of the Association was "to unite all British nurses in membership of a recognised profession and to provide for their registration on terms, satisfactory to physicians and surgeons, as evidence of their having received systematic training"[11]. A three-year period of training was suggested, and possible certification by the Board, who would insist on a minimum standard of professional proficiency.

A General Council was set up with the rather unwieldly composition of "a President and vice-Presidents, 100 medical men, 100 matrons and 100 sisters or nurses'[12]: the constitution was so worded that much power inevitably rested in the hands of members of the London Teaching Hospitals, since the composition of the Executive Committee was the President (Mrs. Fenwick) "the matrons of the London Teaching Hospitals, 14 doctors and 15 other nurses of whom 12 had to be matrons"[13]; their register opened in 1889.

The position was now, that the two rival bodies (The Hospitals' Association and The British Nurses' Association) had each opened their own register of nurses: the principle of some form of registration was quite widely accepted, but the reasons for it differed between the two associations. The Hospitals' Association merely wanted a record of practising nurses for use by doctors, matrons and employing authorities. The British Nurses' Association saw the register as a method of protection for the public and a way of professional recognition for nurses. There is little published evidence that either register was widely used.

In order to achieve their ultimate aim of state registration, the British Nurses' Association needed an Act of Parliament. In 1889, Dr. Fenwick persuaded the British Medical Association to pass a resolution asking for this. There is evidence that Miss Nightingale intervened successfully to prevent it. Her feelings against registration were leading her to spend more and more time opposing it, and many of her friends regretted her absorption in the fight. Jowett* wrote "it is a comparative trifle among all the work you have done"[14].

The attitude of the Hospitals' Association at this time is interesting. In an attempt to assess the situation, they sent a questionnaire to 34 hospitals in England and Scotland "which professed to educate nurses". According to the *Nursing Record*, they subsequently published a report based on 19 replies—some of which were individual opinions—saying that "less than half approved of registration, while the rest desired to be let alone". The President, Dr. Bristowe, stated that as this proved that it was impossible to form a voluntary register, this concluded the connection of the Hospitals' Association with the register of nurses. However, later in the same year, the National Pension Fund for Nurses was incorporated: the articles being signed by Dr. Bristowe, Henry Burdett and others. One of these was "to provide and keep a register for trained and certificated nurses"[15].

Everyone became more and more involved in the battle and neither Mrs. Fenwick nor Henry Burdett lost any opportunity to air their views in (respectively) the *Nursing Record* and *The Hospital*. The *Nursing Record's* comment on a pamphlet against the registration of nurses, published by Mr. Henry

* Benjamin Jowett, Master of Balliol.

Bonham Carter, Secretary of the Nightingale Fund, was that "it contained statements which were not arguments, and arguments which were not relevant"[16]. To protect herself, Mrs. Fenwick threatened Mr. Burdett with legal action if he libelled her in *The Hospital*.

The British Nurses' Association's next step was to obtain a Royal Charter. Queen Victoria's daughter Princess Christian, had been associated with the movement since it started and consented to become its patron. A Charter was granted in 1893 and from then on the British Nurses' Association could use the prefix "Royal". However, the phrase "maintenance and publication of a register of nurses", which had been asked for, was altered so that "register" became "list". It is probable that Miss Nightingale was again behind this. After the Charter had been granted, she signed a letter to *The Times* saying: "the list will have nothing in common with legal Registers of the Medical and other professions, but will simply be a list of nurses published by the Association"[17].

There had also been opposition to the Charter itself: a letter sent to the *Nursing Record* was headed "The Proposed Registration of Nurses—Memorial of Nurse-Training School Authorities" and, referring to the proposed Charter, said that "if the enrolment of nurses in a common register were carried out, it would:

  (i) lower the position of the best trained nurses;

  (ii) be detrimental to the advancement of the teaching of nursing;

  (iii) be disadvantageous to the public; and

  (iv) be injurious to the medical practitioner",

the letter ended by saying that the signatories would "offer, thereto, all legitimate opposition in our power". It was signed by representatives of the following hospitals: St. Thomas's, Guy's, The Westminster, St. Bartholomew's, Charing Cross, King's College, The London, St. Mary's, St. Marylebone Infirmary and St. George's[18]. Despite all opposition however the Charter was granted.

N.B. The reader may wonder why so many references are from the Editorials of the *Nursing Record* of 1893. In 1892 Mrs. Fenwick took over this journal to provide an outlet for her views: most of the Editorials for 1893 are headed "The Registration of Nurses" and give an account of the events of the 1880s.

During the following year, disagreement arose between the Bedford Fenwicks and other members of the now Royal British Nurses' Association, possibly since the Fenwick's highly militant views were too much for their colleagues. Dr. Fenwick resigned as Treasurer and Mrs. Fenwick was not re-elected as President. A certain amount of bitterness developed between the two factions and Mrs. Fenwick sought new channels for her fight for registration. In 1894 she founded the Matrons' Council of Great Britain and Ireland which was pledged to support this ideal. During the next few years discussions continued, but it was not until the turn of the century that events seemed to move towards any solution. In 1899, at a meeting of the Matrons' Council, Mrs. Fenwick successfully proposed the formation of an International Council of Nurses, and at their annual meeting in Buffalo, U.S.A. in 1901 she made a speech reiterating the points nearest to her heart: "all nurses, who have considered the question intelligently, have grasped the fundamental principle that our profession, like every other, needs registration and control: and we claim that this power of control should rest in our own hands, that, in our corporate capacity, we must have the right to live and move and have our being, and that it is from our own ranks that the woman must step out to whom the responsibility of guiding our destines must be entrusted"[19].

The registrationists' hands were strengthened by two events in 1902: first, and most effectively by the passing of the Midwives Registration Act, and secondly by the formation of the Society for the State Registration of Trained Nurses. Two years later this Society amalgamated with the Matrons' Council, the League of St. Bartholomew's Hospital Nurses, and the Leicester Royal Infirmary Nurses' League to form the National Council of Nurses of the United Kingdom. This body was pledged to support the plea for State Registration and continued to represent the nurses of Great Britain at the International Council, until its amalgamation with the Royal College of Nursing in 1963.

During 1903 and 1904, two unsuccessful Bills were presented to Parliament, the first by the Royal British Nurses' Association and the second by the Society for the State Registration of trained nurses. However, their effect was such that in June 1904 Parliament ordered that a Select Committee of the House of

Commons be set up to report on the whole question of the Registration of nurses.

THE SELECT COMMITTEE ON THE REGISTRATION
OF NURSES 1904–1905

On June 24th, 1904 the members of the Select Committee were announced: they were Dr. Robert Ambrose, Major Bagot, Mr. Arthur Henderson, Mr. Charles Hobhouse, Dr. Hutchinson, Viscount Morpeth, Mr. Mount, Mr. Pierpoint, Sir John Stirling Maxwell, Mr. Tennant and Sir John Tuke. They met for the first time on July 7th and during the next year examined witnesses. They also studied written evidence and presented their report to the House of Commons. This was ordered to be printed on July 25th, 1905.

The witnesses examined included, "members of the medical profession, matrons, superintendents of nursing institutions, nurses whose experience has been gained abroad as well as nurses who work in this country, one male nurse, representatives of the Civil Service and lay members of hospital committees"[20].

In 1904 the witnesses who spoke in favour of Registration were Dr. Bedford Fenwick, Miss Margaret Huxley, "who trained at St. Bartholomew's Hospital and has a surgical home in Dublin'[21]; Miss Isla Stewart, Matron of St. Bartholomew's Hospital; Mr. Michael Walsh "the managing director of the Male Nurses (Temperance) Corporation Ltd."[22], who before his appointment to this post ten years previously, had had 17 years in nursing; Miss Annie Hobbs, the Secretary of the Royal British Nurses' Association; and Miss Amy Hughes, Superintendent of the County Nursing Association in affiliation with the Queen Victoria Jubilee Institute for Nurses.

Those opposed were Mr. Charles Burt, Chairman of the Central Hospital Council for London, Chairman of the Board of Governors of the Royal Free Hospital, and a Visitor for the King Edward Hospital Fund for London: Mr. Sidney Holland, "Chairman of The London Hospital, the biggest in England, Chairman of Poplar Hospital which has 100 beds and Chairman of Tilbury Hospital, a cottage hospital"[23] and Dr. Norman Moore a physician at St. Bartholomew's Hospital.

During the course of his evidence Dr. Bedford Fenwick, the spokesman of the "Registration Party", said he had attempted

7

to obtain a Select Committee in 1896. He felt it was essential to have a Council for Registration, Examination, Control and Discipline: there was a great diversity and want of uniformity in hospitals training nurses and "a properly trained nurse ought to be able to undertake the care of any case either surgical or medical"[24]. He felt that at least 40,000 out of 80,000 practising nurses had had no training. Questioned about fees he, "supposed nurses would not mind £5 5s. 0d. for examination and registration"[25] and suggested that the minimum age for examination should be 21 years.

Miss Stewart agreed, in the main, with Dr. Fenwick but felt the age of entry (not examination) should be 21 years. Her main evidence was a description of her own training at the Nightingale School, and the present training at St. Bartholomew's. Miss Stewart went to St. Thomas's as a probationer in 1879 and after eight months "took charge of a ward". She remained there a further six years. At no time was a certificate given but "a receipt was given for good conduct at the end of three years". At St. Bartholomew's the Matron selected those she considered suitable for training and they were then examined in elementary anatomy and physiology by a surgeon and physician (one of them Dr. Norman Moore) and were examined physically. At the end of three months they came before a small committee of Instructors of Nurses (doctors), the Clerk of the Hospital "and me". If the record was good they were appointed probationers for three years. During the first year they had lectures in anatomy and physiology by the Instructors of Nurses, and in nursing by Matron and her assistants: at the end of the first year they were examined in these subjects. If they passed, they continued in training for two years and had weekly lectures from nurses. At the end of three years they were examined again (the pass mark was 50 per cent), and if they passed, they were given a certificate. If they failed they could try again after six months.

Mr. Walsh supported Dr. Fenwick's views on behalf of male nurses and wanted equal opportunities for men and women.

Miss Hobbs told of her training at the West London Hospital ($4\frac{1}{2}$ years). She favoured registration, as she felt there was danger from incompetent and untrained people practising. Questioned on existing nurses, she said "I would put them on the Register by right of what they had done, the certificates which they now hold, and the good characters which they must all be able to give proof of"[26].

For the opposition, Mr. Charles Burt said his Council represented the governing bodies of 12 teaching hospitals and eight other important hospitals in London: presenting the views of the Council he said that they were opposed to State Registration and would oppose any Bill. He submitted a paper which contained over 600 signatures, but added that "Guy's are not with us in this matter"[27]. This list of signatures is given in an appendix to the Select Committee report; they include those of 19 chairmen or treasurers of hospitals, 27 persons holding important appointments in hospital work, 101 surgeons and physicians, over 150 matrons and over 480 nurses. The list of doctors is headed by Lister and includes Patrick Manson: the list of nurses is headed by Eva C. E. Luckes, and the additional signatures include Elizabeth Garrett Anderson. This last is most interesting as Dr. Garrett Anderson spent many years fighting for the recognition of women in medicine.

Mr. Burt handed in a second paper (also in the Appendix) which was headed "re the Royal British Nurses' Association" this paper spoke against the work and views of the Association and its first signature is that of Florence Nightingale.

Mr. Sidney Holland produced lengthy arguments against registration and said that the matrons of every hospital except St. Bartholomew's, Charing Cross and Guy's (Miss Stewart, Miss Heather Bigg and Miss Sarah Swift), were opposed to it. He gave 13 reasons for opposing registration, among them that it would give no safeguard to either the public or the doctors, that nursing could not be tested by examination since "examinations come very easy to some people", and "all a nurse would care about is enough knowledge to be registered"[28]. He said that a "uniform standard" was a very illusory expression and warned the Committee against accepting the views of the Matrons' Council which he said represented only Mrs. Fenwick, Miss Stewart and Miss Heather Bigg. He agreed that doctors and midwives had a Register but said "the analogy is different. The midwife is Registered to go into a special technical job, and it does not matter what her character is, if she can do the job"[29]. Dr. Norman Moore thought there was great danger in having a register of nurses, "that it would lead

9

to the establishment of an imperfectly educated order of medical practitioners"[30]. He thought that examinations by a central body would be less efficient and "that to examine 2,000 nurses a year would be a serious business. Serious and expensive. Question. Very expensive? Answer. Very expensive"[31]. He also felt that if a minimum standard were fixed, the tendency would be to be satisfied with the minimum. This is reminiscent of Miss Nightingale who, in a letter to Henry Bonham Carter (one of the signatories of Mr. Burt's paper) in 1891, wrote: "If you register good and indifferent together, the inferior so largely preponderating, the minimum of qualification will inevitably become the maximum to be aimed at"[32].

Dr. Bedford Fenwick was recalled twice and on his third appearance presented two papers; one set out the position of the Royal British Nurses' Association. The other was headed General Nursing Council.

"Estimate of probable income and expenditure (excluding all receipts from examination fees and expenses of examinations and certificates)".

It laid out a miniature balance sheet. The left hand side was based on 60,000 nurses wanting registration and each paying £2 2s. 0d. (£126,000) and an annual influx of 2,500 persons (£5,250).

The payments side was based on the existing General Medical Council expenses.

   (i) General Medical Council, with 34 members, paid out £4,266 in payments to them.

     If the General Nursing Council had 31 members £5,000 "should be outside the mark".

  (ii) The General Medical Council printing costs etc., were £1,381 19s. 4d.

     So the General Nursing Council should not be more than £2,000.

 (iii) The General Medical Council office expenses were £925 4s. 4d. and legal expenses £235 18s. 2d.

     So adding £500 for rent "it would be safe to estimate that the General Nursing Council expenses under 'office' would not exceed £1,500, and legal expenses would not exceed £200".

	£		£
Dividends on		Payments to members	5,000
£126,000 at 3½%	4,400	Printing, postage and	
Registration fees		stationery	2,000
2,500 at £2 2s. 0d.	5,250	Office expenses	1,500
Sale of publications	50	Legal expenses	200
		Miscellaneous	300
	£9,700		£9,000
		Balance	700
33			£9,700

It is obvious that Dr. Fenwick had given much thought to this and realised that a Registering Council must be a viable financial body. In spite of the bitterness and wrangling in the profession it is cheering to note that he envisaged nurses requiring less legal advice than their medical colleagues!

The Select Committee reassembled during the next Session of Parliament in 1905 and examined the rest of the witnesses. It is not possible to divide all the later witnesses into those for or against Registration since some were called because of their expert knowledge in a specific field.

Four witnesses spoke against State Registration. These were Miss Eva C. E. Luckes, Matron of The London Hospital; Mr. Archer Mobray Upton, Clerk and Solicitor to the Society of Apothecaries; Dr. A. Percy Allen and Dr. W. G. Dickinson, both general practitioners.

Fourteen witnesses spoke for State Registration: these were Miss Christina Forrest, Matron of the Victoria and Bournemouth Nursing Institute and Home Hospital; Miss Ella R. Wortabet who trained at The London Temperance and Middlesex Hospitals, and who had spent many years abroad: Mrs. Fenwick; Miss Lavina Dock, a well known American nurse who trained at Bellevue Hospital, New York; Sir James Crichton-Browne, F.R.S. one of the Lord Chancellor's visitors in Lunacy; Sir Victor Horsley and Mr. Langley Browne, representing the British Medical Association; Dr. William Bezley Thorne, vice-president of the Royal British Nurses' Association; Mr. James Smith Whittaker, M.R.C.S., L.R.C.P., Medical Secretary of the

British Medical Association; Miss Beatrice Kent, who had 13 years' nursing experience in London and the provinces; Dr. Edwin Hyla Greves, a general practitioner; Mr. James Russell Motion, Inspector of Poor and Clerk to the Parish Council of Glasgow; Miss Elizabeth Shannon, Matron of the Western Infirmary, Glasgow; and Lady Helen Munroe Fergusson, vice-president of the Association for the State Registration of Nurses.

Two witnesses would not commit themselves entirely to the idea of State Registration but believed that some form of control was necessary; they were Mrs. Charles Hobhouse, wife of one of the members of the Select Committee who gave evidence as a member of the public, with experience of rural nursing; and Sir Henry Charles Burdett, K.C.B.

The specialist witnesses were Mr. George William Duncan, the administrator for the Central Midwives Board, who gave evidence of experience gained since the Midwives Act and of finance; and Professor Ernest William White, M.B., M.R.C.P., Professor of Psychological Medicine, King's College Hospital, and Dr. G. E. Shuttleworth representing the Asylum Workers' Association, both of whom spoke about mental nursing and the Medico-Psychological Association.

Miss Luckes was the only nurse called who spoke against the need for a Registration Act, and her evidence filled 15 pages of the report—the longest single piece of evidence heard by the committee. She said she had been at The London Hospital for 24 years and that she agreed entirely with the evidence given by Sidney Holland. She thought that State Registration would be "such an injustice to the best nurses and a perfunctory recommendation"[34]. She felt it would make nurses more scientific—which she deplored—and that with the present system it was possible for the training school to give an up-to-date recommendation since it kept in touch with the nurses. She thought it was too early in the nursing profession's history for it to be stereotyped and that anyway, for many cases very little training went a very long way. If a Central Board were set up, anyone actively engaged in nursing would find it impossible to combine work on the Board with doing their own work, and would get out of touch with current opinions.

A large part of Miss Luckes' evidence consisted of a description of the training then given at The London Hospital. Candidates were interviewed, and if healthy and acceptable spent six weeks at the Preliminary Training House (Tredegar House): in the seventh week they were examined in elementary hygiene, elementary physiology, cookery and practical nursing. Those who passed the examination and appeared suitable transferred to the hospital. From then on they had four hours theoretical instruction a week. There were three courses of lectures a year, and the examination, which was set by an outside examiner, consisted of papers, a viva voce and a practical test in the wards. At the end of two years a certificate was given and nurses were appointed either to the hospital staff or to the private nursing staff, according to personal fitness and vacancies.

She quoted figures as follows: 28 fresh candidates were taken into training every seven weeks (about 200 a year), and in the previous ten years a total of 619 nurses had satisfactorily completed the two-year training and received certificates (on average 60 per year).

Asked about the private nursing staff Miss Luckes said "we started our private nursing institution in 1886 to provide nurses for the sick rich, St. Thomas's Hospital having done wonders for the sick poor"[35]. Candidates normally started training at the age of 25 but were occasionally taken at the age of 22 or 23.

Miss Luckes thought a longer course (than two years) would make nurses learn more than is essential for skilled nursing, "which is likely to bring them into conflict with the doctors"[36]. She did not want uniformity of training as she thought that different personalities of nurses were suitable for different types of work, and it would be a waste of time to train all for everything. At The London Hospital, probationers were moved regularly to work in medical, surgical and children's wards, but if a nurse were particularly skilful in one type of case she would be used for this again.

She handed in papers showing the record of theoretical and practical training of a London Hospital probationer, and of her subsequent work on the staff.

Mr. Upton spoke on behalf of the Society of Apothecaries. The Society considered Registration unnecessary and undesirable and thought it would not assist the public, or medical men. If a council were set up, the Society should be represented on it, as representing the general practitioner "who of all medical men is the one who will be most affected"[37]. Asked if Registration would benefit the profession of nurses, he said "that, of course raises the whole principle. The idea, no doubt, is to elevate nursing into a profession just as law or medicine or the church"[38]. He did not think nurses merited that elevation!

The two general practitioners said that the Incorporated Medical Practitioner Association was against Registration. They thought it would be financially unworkable and that if it were compulsory there would not be enough Registered nurses to care for the sick poor. Dr. Dickinson said that Registration was not a burning question amongst the doctors. "A certain number are interested in the matter. I am afraid that the apathy of the medical profession is very great about any matter. A few influential men, of course, can carry anything of that sort without much trouble"[39].

The witnesses who spoke in favour of Registration re-iterated the points made in 1904.

Miss Forrest spoke of the different standards in different hospitals, and how even within the same hospitals standards could change under different officials. She said there was a lack of a general level of education in many hospitals: she was in favour of voluntary Registration and thought that hospitals with 50 beds could be training schools if the training was well organised. She thought a three-year course was essential with both written and practical examinations at the end for which a fee of 1 guinea could be charged. She felt that any Central Board should have the power to strike nurses off the Register in certain cases, and did not want two classes of Registered Nurses. Miss Wortabet favoured higher fees—she thought 3 guineas examination fee and 2 guineas registration fee were permissible. She thought the Council should consist of doctors, matrons and nurses. On being asked "should I be right in thinking that your main object in taking the views you do is that you think your calling ought to be erected into a profession?" she replied "yes"[40].

Mrs. Fenwick agreed with all that had been said by Miss Stewart, Miss Huxley and Miss Forrest. She read a long statement and was questioned on countries which already had Registration; she felt New Zealand was the best. She said: "I claim that there is at present one dead level of mediocrity in the nursing world and under present conditions, as influence counts for so much, it is not always the best qualified women who are appointed to the higher posts in hospitals, especially to the position of matron"[41]. She did not agree that State Registration would make nurses compete with doctors, and felt that friction arose from too little training, not too much. She agreed with Miss Wortabet on the level of fees and did not favour an annual retention fee.

She strongly disapproved of two classes of Registered nurses and spent a long time discussing the current scandals which arose when nurses who were sent to prison could take up their job again after being discharged. She handed in a paper giving details of 89 such cases.

In support of a three-year period of training Mrs. Fenwick produced the following facts:

Of 17 hospitals with 100 or more beds, in London, 16 had a three-year course and one a two-year course. This last refers to The London Hospital, and Mrs. Fenwick pointed out that as two years' service was expected after training, nurses had been working for four years before being available to the public.

Of 55 hospitals with 100 beds or more, in the provinces, 48 had a three-year course, one a four-year training and service programme, three gave a two or three years' certificate and three had a two-year course.

Both of the two Welsh hospitals and all 14 in Scotland (with 100 beds or more) had a three-year course.

In Ireland 11 of the 13 hospitals had a three-year training and two a four year course.

When questioned about the training at The London she explained that when she was there as a sister, the training was three years—not two. She was dissatisfied with the schedule of training handed in by Miss Luckes, and said "that nurse was scurried through 20 wards in 12 months: I do not call that training"[42].

Miss Dock handed in a statement describing developments in the United States of America, where eight States had laws to regulate training and Bills were pending in ten others; in all, Registration was permissive not compulsory. She thought a registration fee of £1 to £2 reasonable. Asked if there was any incidental advantage in legislation being permissive and not compulsory she said "we would not have gotten it. It would have been refused to us"[43].

Sir James Crichton-Browne thought the Register would weed out negligence, stupidity and incompetence and likened the one portal system (one class of Registered Nurse) to the training for medicine. Registration should be a minimum adequate qualification—the best could go on to higher qualifications as doctors did. Asked about competition between nurses and doctors he said "I have always found that it is the uneducated, inferior nurse that presumes"[44].

The doctors who represented the British Medical Association said they agreed that Registration was desirable. Dr. Langley Browne felt that the main opposition to it came from London and said that the British Medical Association represented general practitioners (of which he was one) as well as consultants. Dr. Bezley Thorne said that the Royal British Nurses' Association register was only a stop-gap and would stop when a State Register was established. He handed in a paper giving the Royal British Nurses' Association's answer to the Manifesto. Miss Beatrice Kent, Dr. Greves, Mr. Motion, Miss Shannon and Lady Munroe Fergusson all gave similar views to the previous speakers, differing on detail of fees and as to whether Registration should be compulsory or permissive.

Sir Henry Burdett was called twice and his total evidence covered over 20 pages: although on several occasions he was asked to be brief his statements were lengthy and he handed in three papers.

His views had obviously changed since the 1880's and he now favoured a three-year training. On being asked if nursing had taken a tremendous leap forward in the last ten years he said "yes"—and added that the number who had adopted a three-year training was considerable; "they are obliged to do that; that, I think, must be put down to the credit of Mrs. Bedford Fenwick. To Mrs. Bedford Fenwick is due the credit of insisting upon the three-years' course. She has done a very great work in insisting on that"[45]. This too is a change in viewpoint. Burdett agreed that training schools had no uniform standard. He wanted a Bill providing for registration and inspection of training schools, each of which must provide a recognised training, hold examinations, grant a certificate in a certain form and publish a register each year of all nurses trained and certificated. He said Guy's already did this and was apparently referring to the Nurses' League. He said that at the present time, training schools were self-centred and most of them opposed State Registration. "It is a great pity they do not co-operate"[46].

He felt that a State Register of nurses could never ensure that they would keep up to date, whereas a register of training schools with post-graduate courses would do this.

When he was recalled, Sir Henry Burdett, also gave figures as to the numbers of training schools which approximated closely to Mrs. Fenwick's. Neither of them appear to have included the Poor Law Infirmaries. On being asked his views on the attitude of some of the best schools, he said "the individual idiosyncrasies of managers of a few institutions must not rule against Parliament and the people"[47].

Mrs. Hobhouse spoke from her experience as a member of a Committee of the Rural Nursing Association. Since 1893 this association had 15 nurses on its staff and was organised for philanthropic not financial reasons. She said that the partially trained nurse was competent and well able to cope in rural areas—complicated cases went to hospital. She agreed with State Registration as an ideal, but wanted two classes of nurse so that the rural nurses could do the simple work.

The classification of nurses could be obstetric, medical and surgical, and the rural nurse would not need a surgical qualification. Any examination should be based on a definite curriculum of training and the minimum period of training for the highly trained should be two years. Mrs. Hobhouse felt that the Central Board should be one-third lay members, one-third doctors and one-third nurses.

Mr. Duncan gave evidence about the Central Midwives Board. Its examination fee was 1 guinea and the certificate fee was 10s. The Act was compulsory in that no midwife who was uncertified might claim to be so; the unqualified midwife was free to practise until 1910. The Board could strike midwives off the roll for malpractice, negligence, misconduct or breach of the rules.

Professor White and Dr. Shuttleworth described the work of the Medico-Psychological Association in detail.

The Association was formed in 1841 and had a system of training and examination for mental nurses. Its regulations were:
(1) There was a probationary period of three months.
(2) There was a three-year training including the probationary period which must be completed before the examination and held in not more than two institutions.
(3) The Council of the Medico-Psychological Association recognised institutions for training.

The system of training included:
(1) Lectures and demonstrations by medical men—12 a year of which 75 per cent must be attended.
(2) Clinical instruction in the wards by doctors.
(3) Exercises under senior nurses.
(4) Study of the handbook of the Medico-Psychological Association—drawn up in 1884.
(5) Periodic examinations—one each year.
(6) Scope of training laid down.

A schedule of training had to be filled in and submitted to the Registrar, four weeks before the examination, signed by the superintendent of the hospital. The examination included written papers, viva and practical.

Professor White thought the system was excellent and would work for other nurses—the examination fee was 5s. He thought £1 fee to be enough and felt a three-year training was necessary.

In the Committees' report to the House of Commons there were 26 recommendations, the majority of which were concerned with the registration of nurses. It was felt, generally, that there should be some change in the conditions under which nursing was carried on, and that this was both desirable and practicable. The Committee found that although the majority of training schools wanted change, they could not agree on how this should be achieved.

Recommendation 11 read "your Committee are agreed that it is desirable that a Register of Nurses should be kept by a Central Body appointed by the State and that, while it is not desirable to prohibit unregistered persons from nursing for gain, no persons should be entitled to assume the designation of 'Registered Nurse' whose name is not upon the Register"[48].

The suggested Constitution of the Central Body was that it

should consist of matrons, nurses and representatives of the medical profession, of training schools for nurses and of the public; a membership of 11–15 was thought to be best.

Other recommendations referred to existing nurses, to the recognition, approval and inspection of training schools, and to the conduct of examinations which were to be held at, and by, the training schools. While agreeing that a three-year training was desirable the Committee felt that the length should not be laid down by Act of Parliament, but decided by the Central Body. A Registration fee not exceeding 1 guinea was recommended.

Recommendation 21 suggested that four years after the Central Body was set up, they should report to the Privy Council on the desirability of "a separate Register of nurses whose training is of a lower standard than that laid down for the Register of Nurses"[49].

The publication of the Report gave great satisfaction to the Registrationists who would have been justified in believing that a Nurses Act was at last in sight. It is surprising, however, that no action was taken by the Government. The Select Committee has been described in great detail since most of the arguments for and against registration were exactly the same in 1904 and 1919, and in reading the eventual Registration Act one can see clearly that the Select Committees' work and Report were not wasted: indeed, anyone familiar with nursing politics today, may see the roots of some of our practices and problems in the evidence of the witnesses in 1904-5.

For the next few years Registration Bills were regularly introduced and kept before the House of Commons, and according to Mrs. Fenwick, writing in the *British Journal of Nursing*,* were "blocked, night after night by representatives of nursing schools, the Hon. Harry Levi Lawson (later Lord Burnham) as a member of the Committee of The London, popping up and objecting"[50]. She also implied that certain sections of the Press took a leading part in "downing the nurses".

In 1908 Lord Balfour of Burleigh introduced a Bill in the House of Lords to provide for an official directory of nurses. Sir Henry Burdett described it as a "damned bad Bill"[51] and it was defeated by 20–53. Early in the same year a Bill brought by the Society for The State Registration of Trained Nurses was

* Previously the *Nursing Record*.

introduced, again in the Lords, and had a second reading on July 6th; it was passed with the support of the Government on November 10th, and on November 16th it was brought to the House of Commons and ordered to be printed. However, Mr. Asquith (the then Prime Minister) refused to give time for its consideration. Also in 1908 the Scottish nurses organised a Registration Committee. In 1909 three unsuccessful Bills were introduced, and the Registrationists must have been feeling desperate. In 1910, Mrs. Fenwick invited all interested organisations to meet to form the Central Committee for the State Registration of Nurses: the organisations concerned were: The British Medical Association, The Royal British Nurses' Association, The Matrons' Council, the Society for the State Registration of Trained Nurses, the Fever Nurses' Association, the Irish Nurses' Association, the Scottish Nurses' Association and the Association for the Promotion of the Registration of Nurses in Scotland; these were later joined by the National Union of Trained Nurses. It was also in 1910 that Miss Florence Nightingale, O.M. died, at the age of 90. In 1910, 1911, 1912 and 1913 the Central Committee presented Bills to Parliament and these, according to the *British Journal of Nursing* were "persistently blocked by the Central Hospital Council, led by The London and St. Thomas's"[52].

Early in 1914 another Bill was introduced in the House of Commons. In one of the national newspapers Dr. Edward Wilberforce Goodall, one of the Honorary Secretaries of the Central Committee, was quoted as saying, "the arguments in support of the Bill are unanswerable, and there is no reasonable ground for opposing it. There are three main points which the Bill seeks to establish. We want:

(1) Minimum of three years' training in a recognised training school for nurses.

(2) A General Nursing Council, on which nurses will be well represented, to control the examination of nurses.

(3) Every trained nurse to pass the same examination before being registered as a trained nurse.

There is a more urgent need for registration than there was a few years ago, for owing to the wonderful advances in doctoring, and to the development of hospitals, many more nurses are required, while the competition of other callings has caused

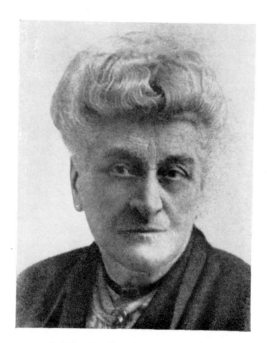

1. Mrs. E. G. Fenwick, S.R.N. 1.

ABC OF STATE REGISTRATION

A   is the Act which we hope to see passed

B   is the Bill we must nail to the mast

C   is our Charter of Liberty free

D   for the Doctors who with it agree

E   for the Eager who work till they drop

F   is the Freedom which bears such a crop

G   for the Growth of professional rule

H   for our Hospital and Training School

I   the Ideal which each nurse desires

J   for the Journal that high aims inspires

K   for the Keeness the nursing world needs

L   for our Leaders we thank for their deeds

M   for the Matron of each training school

N   for the Nurse who respects her wise rule

O   the 'One Portal' through which we must pass

P   is the Pro. who fails sometimes, alas

Q   is the Quest we have sought to obtain

R   for the Register we shall soon gain

S   for the Slacker who's naught but a curse

T   for the Title of Registered Nurse

U   for the Uniform we must protect

V   for the Voters who Council elect

W   the Wards where the nurses find scope

X   for the Exam not too hard we hope

Y   for the Years of spade work on the Bill

Z   for the Zealous who work at it still

Violetta Thurstan,
British Journal of Nursing
May 6th, 1916

2. An ABC of registration.

fewer nurses to be available. . . . There is no encouragement for women to enter the profession, because anyone can call herself a trained nurse, and there is no recognised standard. . . . The names of some matrons of hospitals have been cited as opponents to the scheme, but we have more than 500 matrons— the great majority—on our side, and the opinion of those formally opposed to us is rapidly changing. . . . But why should anyone oppose the Registration of Nurses when it is thought necessary to register doctors, dentists, lawyers, chemists, midwives and plumbers?"[53]. (Dr. Goodall was later to be a vocal member of the first General Nursing Council for England and Wales.) Assessment of numerical membership of any group is always difficult, and if one accepts the figures given by the opposing sides for the numbers of matrons in either camp at this time (457 against—500 for)[54], then there were obviously more matrons than hospitals!

This latest Bill was introduced under the ten-minute rule and for the first time a Division was challenged and produced a majority vote of 228. Mrs. Fenwick's comment was, "I was the only nurse in the House during this historic event, and was only saved from whirling down the marble steps in my excitement by being caught round the waist by Dr. Chapple (M.P.), and thereby no doubt saved a serious accident. One cannot step on air with impunity".[55] However, her excitement was premature as little progress was made: world events overtook local considerations and when the Great War started in August 1914, Private Members ceased to promote legislation by order of the Government.

THE COLLEGE OF NURSING

For two years there was no mention of registration, but in 1916 a new force emerged. Mrs. Fenwick's supporters had never included the majority of the London teaching hospital matrons, and she had not been a matron herself for 29 years. A new generation had grown up in the profession, who chose to link themselves with the hospital administrators—and a feeling grew of the need for some form of professional association with wider aims than the one target of State Registration. The prime movers were Miss Sarah Swift who was now in charge of the nurses' department of the British Red Cross Society, the Hon.

Arthur Stanley, Chairman of the British Section of the Red Cross, Mr. Cooper Perry, Medical Superintendent of Guy's, Miss Rachael Cox-Davies, Matron of the Royal Free Hospital, Miss Alicia Lloyd Still, Matron of St. Thomas's Hospital and Mr. Comyns Berkeley, Consultant at the Middlesex Hospital. These six were to found the College of Nursing Ltd., which came into being on March 27th, 1916. The principal objects of the College were stated as being:

(1) To promote the better education and training of nurses and the advancement of nursing as a profession in all or any of its branches.

(2) To promote uniformity of curriculum.

(3) To recognise and approve training schools.

(4) To make and maintain a register of persons to whom certificates of proficiency, or of training and proficiency had been granted.

(5) To promote Bills in Parliament for any object connected with the interests of the nursing profession and, in particular, with nurse education, organisation, protection, or for their recognition by the State.

There was an immediate response to a circular letter sent out by the Hon. Arthur Stanley which went to the training schools and other interested bodies; but the Central Committee for State Registration were not enthusiastic. Many of its members felt that it was not in the best interests of the nursing profession since it by-passed the need for legal recognition. They also felt a sense of some injustice since they had agreed to discontinue efforts to achieve a Nurses Act for the duration of the war.

Mrs. Fenwick wrote "what time, therefore, more indefensible for those who for years have opposed every effort of the conjoint professions of medicine and nursing to organise the education and discipline of trained nurses"[56]. However her main dislike of the new organisation was due to the strong influence of its "lay" backers.

Although State Registration was not among the declared aims of the College of Nursing, within one month of its foundation, Stanley wrote to the Central Committee, inviting them to appoint nine delegates to meet a sub-committee of the Council of the College (also nine), "with the object of coming to an agreement upon the terms of a Bill to be brought before Parliament, as an agreed Bill, at as early a date as possible"[57]. The Central Committee agreed, provided the Bill to be discussed was their own, which was still before Parliament. Although for a few months attempts to achieve unity were made by all interested parties, these failed entirely and by July 1916 there was as much difference of opinion as there had ever been, particularly on the proposed constitution of the General Nursing Council.

The Central Committee said (speaking of the College of Nursing): "such lay organisations are not qualified, neither do they attempt to dominate the General Medical Council. Why, therefore, should they assume control on the General Nursing Council?"[58]. Sir Henry Burdett, writing in *The Hospital*, accused Mrs. Bedford Fenwick of being "the one woman who wishes to keep everything in her own hands and to hold that position by denouncing much that is self respecting and worthy in the nursing world"[59].

By the end of the year the Central Committee and the College of Nursing had each decided to concentrate on their own Bills. In November 1916 Major Chapple, at Question Time in the House of Commons asked the Prime Minister when he would bring in a Registration Bill. The Prime Minister replied: "this is a highly controversial proposal, as my Hon. friend is aware and I cannot, at the present time, undertake to introduce it"[60].

In the next three years a change took place in the politicians' attitude to women's rights and to the views of nurses. Nurses had worked hard throughout the war in trying and difficult circumstances, and as at the end of the Crimean War, the country was grateful. Also women were to get the vote, and no party could afford to ignore a large section of the public on whom they would rely in future for political support. Two comments from the House of Lords in 1919 were "women now have the vote: they have to be considered more than they used to be . . . women are now likely to get what they insist on having," and "if you force nurses to form trades unions in order to secure that which they regard, and rightly regard, as a measure of justice and a right to them, you will simply throw them into the arms of the Labour Party"[61].

Early in 1919 an M.P., Major Barnett, was lucky in the ballot to introduce a Private Members Bill. He "gave it to the nurses' and on March 11th introduced the Central Committee's Bill in the Commons. At first the College of Nursing agreed to support the Bill, in the interests of State Registration[62], and it had a second reading on March 28th. However in the committee stage difficulties arose, due to the many amendments proposed. It appears that the constitution of the General Nursing Council was again a problem, since an Editorial of the *Nursing Times* at this time was headed "The Boomerang" and deplored the weakness of the College representatives in not pressing its case hard enough and being prepared to settle for only four seats![63] By the third reading of the Bill, in June, there were 61 amendments, 12 in the name of the original proposer, Major Barnett. By this time the College had withdrawn its support and introduced a Bill of its own in the House of Lords. Lord Knutsford (Sidney Holland) was quoted in the *Daily Graphic* as saying "a Machiavellian critic could not wish anything better than that the Commons Bill should pass, because it reduces the whole thing to such a ghastly farce that nobody would register. I am going to ask the House of Lords to pass Lord Goschen's Bill (the College Bill) rather than the one that has gone through the Committee stage of the House of Commons, because the latter is brought forward by people who are not representative of nursing at all"[64].

The Lords Bill also achieved a second reading, but in July the Minister of Health, Dr. Addison, asked both sides to withdraw their Bills, and although Major Barnett refused and protested at the delay, no agreement had been reached when the House adjourned in July. In the Autumn session of Parliament, Dr. Addison introduced his own Bill on November 6th and it had a second reading on November 22nd. At a meeting the same month Mrs. Fenwick "as an old war horse and leader" proposed that a vote of thanks should go to Dr. Addison from the meeting: the proposal was carried nem con.[65]

The Bill was finally passed in December and "thanks to the courtesy of the Marquess of Lincolnshire, crimson benches of the Lords were placed at the disposal of women who had accomplished this far-reaching national reform, and nothing can minimise the thrill of emotion and delight experienced by the trained nurses whose high privilege it was to be present on this historic occasion, when with dignified ceremonial, the King's will was proclaimed in the quaint old Norman French—"le Roy le veult"—in which the three Nurses Registration Acts received the Royal Assent"[66].

References

1. A General History of Nursing, p. 260. Seymer.
2. *Nursing Record*—22.3.1893.
3. Ibid.
4. Ibid.
5. Ibid.
6. A History of the Nursing Profession, p. 62. Abel Smith.
7. *Nursing Record*—22.3.1893.
8. The London, p. 105/6. Clarke-Kennedy.
9. Florence Nightingale, p. 570. Woodham Smith.
10. *Nursing Record*—9.3.1893.
11. Ibid.
12. A History of the Nursing Profession, p. 69. Abel Smith.
13. Ibid.
14. Florence Nightingale, p. 572. Woodham Smith.
15. *Nursing Record*—16.3.1893.
16. Ibid—30.3.1893.
17. A History of the Nursing Profession, p. 72. Abel Smith.
18. *Nursing Record*—30.3.1893.
19. A History of Nursing, p. 170. Stewart and Austin.
20. Select Committee on Registration of Nurses, 1904.
21. Ibid.
22. Ibid.
23. Ibid.
24. Ibid.
25. Ibid.
26. Ibid.
27. Ibid.
28. Ibid.
29. Ibid.
30. Ibid.
31. Ibid.
32. Florence Nightingale's Nurses, p. 112. Seymer.
33. Select Committee on Registration of Nurses 1904.
34. Ibid. 1905.
35. Ibid.
36. Ibid.
37. Ibid.
38. Ibid.
39. Ibid.
40. Ibid.

41. Ibid.
42. Ibid.
43. Ibid.
44. Ibid.
45. Ibid.
46. Ibid.
47. Ibid.
48. Ibid.
49. Ibid.
50. *British Journal of Nursing*—22.9.23.
51. Ibid.
52. Ibid—20.10.23.
53. *Daily Express*—6.5.14.
54. A History of the Nursing Profession, p. 82. Abel Smith.
55. *British Journal of Nursing*—20.10.23.
56. Ibid—12.2.16.
57. Ibid—22.4.16.
58. Ibid—22.7.16.
59. A History of the Nursing Profession, p. 91. Abel Smith.
60. *British Journal of Nursing*—11.11.16.
61. A History of the Nursing Profession, p. 93. Abel Smith.
62. *Nursing Times*—28.3.19.
63. Ibid—19.4.19.
64. Ibid—31.5.19.
65. Ibid—8.11.19.
66. *British Journal of Nursing*—17.11.23.

Chapter 2

THE NURSES REGISTRATION ACT 1919

"In 1919, the battle for State Registration was won and past
controversies were forgotten in a very general satisfaction."
MARY STOCKS

It was necessary for Parliament to pass three separate Registration Acts, one for England and Wales, one for Scotland and
one for Ireland (at this time still one country); this was because
each had a separate Ministry of Health. Copies of the 1919 Act
can still be obtained, but it is no longer in force.

The Act, for England and Wales, was a very short document,
covering less than six pages: it had nine Sections in which it
stated that:

1. "There shall be a General Nursing Council for England
and Wales, which shall be a body corporate, by that name, with
perpetual succession and a common seal with power to acquire
and hold land without licence in mortmain."

2. A Register of Nurses was to be formed and kept with five
parts:

(*a*) A general part containing the names of all nurses who
satisfy the conditions of admission to that part of the
Register;

(*b*) a supplementary part containing the names of male
nurses;

(*c*) a supplementary part containing the names of nurses
trained in the nursing and care of persons suffering from
mental diseases;

(*d*) a supplementary part containing the names of nurses
trained in the nursing of sick children;

(*e*) any other prescribed part.

3. The Council were to make rules regulating its work with
regard to the Register, examinations, discipline, its meetings
and committees and the uniform and badge. It was to lay down
conditions of training and the rules for the registration of
'existing' nurses.

This last was to prove one of the most controversial aspects
of the first Council's work and it is important to note the wording of the Act on this point. Rules were to be made "enabling

persons who, within a period of two years after the date on which the rules to be made under the provisions of this paragraph first come into operation, make an application in that behalf (in this Act referred to as 'an existing nurses application') to be admitted to the Register on producing evidence to the satisfaction of the Council that they are of good character, are of the prescribed age, are persons who were for at least three years before the first day of November 1919, bona fide engaged in practice as nurses in attendance on the sick under conditions which appear to the Council to be satisfactory for the purposes of this provision and have adequate knowledge and experience of the nursing of the sick."

The rules were to be approved by the Minister of Health and laid before the House of Commons for 21 days.

Section 4 was concerned with the Council's staff and expenses and Section 5 with the fees to be charged. These last were to be decided by the Council, but in the case of existing nurses the registration fee was not to exceed 1 guinea and the annual retention fee was not to exceed two shillings and sixpence.

Section 6 was concerned with the registration of persons trained outside the United Kingdom, and Section 7 with the procedure to be followed "by any person aggrieved by the removal of his name from the Register" or "by the refusal of the Council to approve an Institution" (for training).

Section 8 dealt with the penalties for the misuse of the title of Registered Nurse, and Section 9 said that the Act only referred to England and Wales.

The Schedule, at the end of the Act, laid down the Constitution of the Council.

There were to be 25 members; for the first Council:

2 were to be appointed by the Privy Council and were to be in no way connected with medicine or nursing;

2 were to be appointed by the Board of Education;

5 were to be appointed by the Minister of Health; and

16 were to be nurses, appointed by the Minister, "after consultation with the Central Committee for the State Registration of Nurses, the College of Nursing, the Royal British Nurses' Association and such other associations or organised bodies of nurses or matrons as represent to the Minister that they desire to be consulted in the matter"[1].

The term of office of the first Council was to be not less than two and not more than three years from the date of the passing of the Act (December 23rd, 1919), and at the end of that time a new Council would come into being with the same composition, except that the 16 nurses were to be elected by nurses who had registered by the time the election was held. After the first Council, members would hold office for five years.

* * *

While the Minister was consulting interested parties about nominees for the first Council, nurses generally rejoiced. A service of thanksgiving was held for the passing of the Nurses Registration Act, in St. Martin in the Fields, on January 23rd, 1920, and the church was packed. Both the Royal British Nurses' Association and the College of Nursing had celebration meetings, and Dr. Addison, tactfully, attended both. According to the *British Journal of Nursing*, the former was the more successful "since it was attended mainly by nurses"[2]. At the College "party" the Minister said, "In regard to the first Register, it was bound to contain the names of a large number of nurses who had practised their profession for a long time, but might not have had the opportunities required in the latest curriculum of training"[3].

Mrs. Fenwick went to the Ministry of Health on several occasions, and according to her own reminiscences, tried hard to ensure that the first Chairman of the General Nursing Council should be a nurse—but she was unsuccessful.

The list of the names of the members of the General Nursing Council for Scotland was the first to be published. Later, on May 1st, 1920, the *British Journal of Nursing* published a "Who's who on the General Nursing Council" (for England and Wales)[4].

The Chairman was to be Mr. J. C. Priestley, K.C., who was called to the Bar in 1888 and in 1906 became a J.P. for Hertfordshire.

The other non-nurse members were:

Lady Hobhouse, wife of the Rt. Hon. Sir Charles Hobhouse, who as Mrs. Charles Hobhouse gave evidence before the Select Committee in 1905; she had been Chairman, Secretary and Treasurer of the Wiltshire Rural Nursing Association.

The Hon. Mrs. Eustice Hills, Chairman of the Council of the National Society of Day Nurseries.

Miss Margaret Janson Tuke, M.A., Principal of Bedford College for Women, University of London.

Rev. G. B. Cronshaw, Chairman and Treasurer, the Radcliffe Infirmary and County Hospital, Oxford.

Sir Thomas Jenner Verrall, M.R.C.S., Consultant Surgeon, Sussex County Hospital, who among his many associations was direct representative of the General Medical Council and delegate of the B.M.A. on the Central Committee for the State Registration of Nurses.

Dr. E. W. Goodall, O.B.E., M.D., Medical Superintendent of the North Western Hospital, Hampstead, and Hon. Medical Secretary of the Central Committee for the State Registration of Nurses since 1910.

Dr. A. Bostock Hill, M.D., Medical Officer of Health for Warwickshire.

Dr. Bedford Pierce, M.D., F.R.C.P., Medical Superintendent of the Retreat, York.

The nurse members were:

Mrs. Ethel Bedford Fenwick.

Miss Alicia Lloyd Still, C.B.E., R.R.C., Matron and Superintendent of the Nightingale Training School, St. Thomas's Hospital, and member of the Council of the College of Nursing Ltd.

Miss Rachael Annie Cox-Davies, R.R.C., Matron of the Royal Free Hospital, who trained at St. Bartholomew's Hospital, and who was a member of the Council of the College of Nursing Ltd.

Miss Margaret Elwin Sparshott, C.B.E., R.R.C., Lady Superintendent of the Royal Infirmary, Manchester, and a member of the Council of the College of Nursing Ltd., who trained at Nottingham General Hospital.

Miss A. Dowbiggin, C.B.E., R.R.C., Matron of Edmonton Union Infirmary, a member of the Matron's Council of Gt. Britain and of the executive of the National Union of Trained Nurses, who trained at Leeds General Infirmary.

Miss C. Seymour Yapp, Matron of Ashton-under-Lyne Poor Law Infirmary, and the author of three textbooks for nurses, who trained at Aston Union Infirmary.

Miss Agnes Mary Coulton, Lady Superintendent of the East

London Hospital for Children, who trained at Guy's Hospital.

Miss Constance Worsley, Matron of the Infirmary for Children, Myrtle Street, Liverpool, who trained at Addenbrookes Hospital.

Miss Susan A. Villiers, Matron of the South Western Hospital, treasurer and vice-president of the Matron's Council, member of the executive and Council of the Royal British Nurses' Association, member of the executive of the National Union of Trained Nurses and a delegate of the Fever Nurses Association to the Central Committee, who trained at St. Bartholomew's Hospital.

Miss Annie McWillie Peterkin, General Superintendent of the Queen Victoria Jubilee Institute for Nurses, and a member of the Council of the College of Nursing Ltd., who trained at Chalmers Hospital, Edinburgh.

Miss Ellinor Smith, Superintendent for Wales of the Queen Victoria Jubilee Institute for Nurses who trained at Sunderland General Hospital.

Miss Isobel Macdonald, Secretary of the Royal British Nurses' Association, and author of a book on home nursing, who trained at the Royal Infirmary, Edinburgh.

Miss Emily Constance Swiss, a health visitor, who trained at the Royal Infirmary, Sheffield.

Miss Alice Cattell, engaged in private nursing and a member of the Royal British Nurses' Association executive committee, who trained at St. George's Hospital.

Miss Maude MacCallum, the Hon. secretary of the Professional Union of Trained Nurses, who trained at Adelaide Hospital, Dublin.

Mr. Tom Christian, M.P.A., a charge nurse at Banstead Hospital, who had trained there.

Of the non-nurses, two were members of the Central Committee. It is difficult to decide whether the College or the Central Committee started with an advantage on the Council, since five nurses clearly had allegiance to each. One historian states that "the College of Nursing had become indisputably the spokesman for the profession"[5] but this is not entirely justified as some members (e.g. Miss MacCullum) belonged both to the College and to one of the organisations associated with the

Central Committee. What is clear is that the Minister had taken considerable pains to ensure that most sectional interests—fever, psychiatric, paediatric, public health, private, male nurses etc., were represented on the General Nursing Council. While this is a most commendable principle, it does not make for harmonious and united efforts, since each representative may spend much energy in preserving the rights of the minority group.

It will be seen that the first, or Caretaker, Council had a formidable task ahead. They had to frame rules which, when approved, would enable existing nurses to register during the two-year "period of grace" in sufficient numbers to provide an electorate. As the period of grace could not start until the rules were approved and as the dissolution of the first Council had to take place at the latest by December 1922, it is obvious that the rules had to be drafted quickly.

HISTORICAL BACKGROUND

The task facing the first General Nursing Council must be considered against the social, political and historical background.

The development of English hospitals

The dissolution of the monasteries (1536–1539) by Henry VIII left England without any hospital system, and with one or two notable exceptions this state of affairs continued for nearly 200 years. However, during the eighteenth century an increasing awareness of the needs of the sick poor, led to an extraordinary development in hospital building. Most of the new hospitals were general hospitals which were built and supported entirely by voluntary contributions. Among them were the following: Bristol Infirmary, 1737; Devon and Exeter Hospital, 1743; Gloucester Infirmary, 1745; Manchester Infirmary, 1752; Leeds Infirmary, 1767; The Radcliffe Infirmary, Oxford, 1770; Leicester Infirmary, 1771; and in London, Westminster Hospital, 1719; Guy's Hospital, 1725; St. George's Hospital, 1733; The London Hospital, 1740; and The Middlesex Hospital, 1745. Many of these were later allowed to bear the title "Royal".

The voluntary hospital system, while producing a much needed service, could not cope adequately with the whole problem—for example by 1861 there were 11,000 patients in voluntary hospitals but over 50,000 sick people in the workhouses[6].

Most of the workhouses had been established following the Poor Law Amendment Act of 1834—but they were never intended to provide specific treatment for the sick, simply accommodation for all those in need, including the destitute, orphans, elderly, widows and mentally ill.

In 1866 and 1875 two further Acts permitted Local Authorities to establish general hospitals; London took the lead in this and was slowly copied by the rest of the country—three of the first local authority hospitals being in Barry, Bradford and Willesden[7].

The nineteenth century was also the age of the development of specialised hospitals and more than 170 were built—many by local authorities—to care for those who needed special treatment or who could not be accommodated in the general hospitals. These were patients with diseases of the eyes, chest, ear, nose and throat, heart and lungs, skin, and also for women, children, incurables, accident victims and those suffering from cancer, fevers, smallpox, paralysis and epilepsy, and stone[8]. This peculiarly English development was to lead to many problems of specialised branches of nursing.

By the early years of the twentieth century some 40,000 patients were being treated in voluntary hospitals and about 100,000 were under the care of the local authorities.

The special care of the mentally ill developed in the nineteenth century although some voluntary institutions existed before this. In 1823 only nine counties had asylums, the largest in Wakefield, for 250 patients and the smallest for 50 patients in Lincoln. A Select Committee set up in 1827 to "consider the state of pauper lunatics in the metropolis", resulted in two Acts of Parliament; one dealt with improvements to the County asylums and the other set up the Metropolitan Commissioners in Lunacy. The next few years saw an increase in the number of County Asylums, the largest being the Middlesex Asylum at Hanwell, with 1,000 patients.

By 1845 there were 18 county asylums, 12 voluntary hospitals and 136 licensed houses which between them provided care for rather less than half the 21,000 people recorded as being insane[9].

The Act of 1845 made the provision of asylums compulsory on the county and principal borough authorities and in the next 20 years a large number of asylums were built with between 500–800 beds[10].

During the nineteenth century a total of 20 Acts of Parliament were passed dealing with the institutional care of the mentally ill. These were finally consolidated in the Lunacy Act of 1890 and the Mental Defectives Act of 1913—which both remained virtually unchanged until the Act of 1959[11].

By 1900 there was accommodation in the mental hospitals for over 80,000 patients.

When the 1919 Nurses Registration Act was passed there were four distinct groups of hospitals. First the voluntary hospitals with a history and tradition extending back nearly 200 years. Second, the Poor Law Hospitals, caring for more than twice as many patients—few with a history of more than 50 years and varying widely in size, resources and standards. Third the "Special" hospitals—some voluntary and some municipal—and generally rather small; and fourth the hospitals for the mentally ill—large, situated in isolated areas, feared by most of the community, and still custodial rather than curative.

The Nursing Service

When one reads the history of any of our great voluntary hospitals, one is struck by the fact that at the beginning little planning or provision was made for any sort of nursing service. The hospital was usually founded by one man or group of men who were eager to provide accommodation and medical treatment, but who considered actual attendants on the sick to be less important. Only as the hospital developed, were nurses appointed. The following figures from a London teaching hospital emphasise this point.

1719 Matron and 1 nurse appointed.
1733 Matron and 1 nurse.
1734 15 beds, 2 nurses.
1735 35 beds, 4 nurses.
1745 86 beds, 11 nurses.
1791 86 beds, 12 nurses.
1800 90 beds, 10 nurses.
1839 106 beds, 16 nurses.
1880 190 beds, 26 nurses and up to 25
     probationers[12].

As is well known, the middle of the nineteenth century saw the beginning of organised nurse training; for the first 20 years the movement was largely confined to the voluntary hospitals. Once training started, the role of the nurse began to emerge and in some cases an attempt was made to separate nursing from domestic work. In 1857 "scrubbers" were employed at St. Bartholomew's Hospital, London, and in 1868 Guy's Hospital followed suit[13].

Before nurse training was established, those who undertook the care of the sick were of the domestic servant class; after 1860 and the opening of the Nightingale Training School, nursing gradually began to be looked on as an acceptable vocation for women with more education and from more wealthy families. The impact of the movement for the emancipation of women, the suffragettes and the 1914–18 war, resulted in a large number of women entering nurse training, especially in the voluntary hospitals.

By 1901 the ratio of nurses to patients in the London teaching hospitals was 1 to 2 or 3, but over half of these were probationers[14]. In the Poor Law Hospitals very different conditions prevailed. Traditionally the sick in the workhouses were cared for by able bodied paupers, and until the end of the nineteenth century few women with training were employed as nurses, since the workhouse masters were unwilling to delegate their authority and conditions were unattractive[15].

In 1897 an order issued by the Local Government Board stated that pauper inmates were no longer to perform the duties of nurse, and that superintendent nurses were to be employed in all workhouses having a nursing staff of three or more; these superintendents could only be nurses who had three years training in a recognised nursing school[16]. This order obviously increased the need for nurses, and many Poor Law Hospitals introduced their own training schools. In 1902 the staff in one Poor Law Hospital with 150 beds for the sick, had a matron, a superintendent nurse, three charge nurses, three assistant nurses, two probationers and one midwifery nurse[17].

In the 20 years 1893–1913 the number of nurses employed in Poor Law Institutions increased from under 3,000 to 7,652[18]. Even so the ratio of nurses to patients in 1901 was 1 to 20[19].

The specialist hospitals developed their own nurse training

35

schemes but had problems with recruitment, especially in the rural areas. Nurses trained in these hospitals had difficulty in finding employment outside their own speciality and in some cases affiliated training schemes were started between specialist and general hospitals.

In the mental hospitals, the position was influenced by the Acts of Parliament passed during the nineteenth century and by the formation of the Medico-Psychological Association in 1841. The movement for special training for mental nurses originated in Scotland and by 1888 classes were being held at Haywards Heath, Dundee, York and Morpeth[20]. However, difficulties in recruiting staff of the right character were encountered since the asylum service expanded so rapidly and the demand was too great[21]. The Medico-Psychological Association (M.P.A.) published a handbook for mental nurses in 1885 which has been continued to this day. By 1905 the M.P.A. were able to report a satisfactory scheme of training to the Select Committee of the House of Commons but the numbers of those in training remained far too few. Traditionally the male and female patients in mental hospitals have always been completely separated and each were cared for by nurses of their own sex. Before 1919 the bulk of male nurses worked in the mental institutions and these were the only places where they had any hope of promotion.

The position in 1919

As already stated, the Minister's appointments to the first General Nursing Council reflected most sectional interests—fever, psychiatric, paediatric, public health, private, male nurses, voluntary and Poor Law hospitals. It is, however of interest to note that of the 16 nurse members, 14 had trained in voluntary hospitals, ten of which were associated with medical schools. Their views on recruitment, training and examinations could not fail to be coloured by this background.

References

1. Nurses Registration Act, 1919.
2. *British Journal of Nursing*—24.1.20.
3. Ibid.
4. Ibid—1.5.20.
5. A History of the Nursing Profession, p. 102. Abel Smith.

6. The Hospitals, p. 46. Abel Smith.
7. The Story of England's Hospitals, pp. 111-112. Courtney Dainton.
8. Ibid.
9. Ibid, pp. 159-161.
10. The History of Mental Nursing, p. 7. Alexander Walk.
11. Trends in the National Health Service, pp. 185–98. Ed. by Farndale.
12. Westminster Hospital, p. 79. Humble and Hansell.
13. The Story of England's Hospitals, p. 118. Courtney Dainton.
14. A History of the Nursing Profession, p. 52. Abel Smith.
15. The Hospitals, p. 210. Abel Smith.
16. Ibid, p. 213. Abel Smith.
17. The Central Middlesex Hospital, p. 37. Allan Gray.
18. The Hospitals, p. 235. Abel Smith.
19. A History of the Nursing Profession, p. 52. Abel Smith.
20. The History of Mental Nursing, p. 11. Alexander Walk.
21. Ibid, p. 7.

Chapter 3

THE CARETAKER COUNCIL (1)

"A house divided against itself cannot stand."
St. Mark, Ch. 3, v. 25

The General Nursing Council for England and Wales met for the first time on Tuesday, May 11th, 1920. Twenty members were present; the absentees were Lady Hobhouse, Dr. Bostock Hill, Mrs. Eustice Hills, Miss Tuke and Miss Seymour Yapp. Having, as yet, no permanent offices or staff, a room and secretary were placed at their disposal at the Ministry of Health. At this meeting it was decided that for the time being business should be in private and reporters excluded. The second resolution was to set up a temporary committee to draw up rules for summoning and regulating meetings of committees and of the Council and to decide the quorum. The same committee was to take steps to find a Registrar, who was to be a woman and a fully trained nurse. The members of this committee were Mrs. Fenwick, Miss Cox-Davies, Dr. Goodall, Miss Macdonald, Miss Sparshott and Mr. Priestley, the Chairman of Council. A Finance Committee was appointed to consider the salary of the Registrar—which members thought should be not less than £550 p.a.—and to find a permanent home for the Council. This committee consisted of Sir Jenner Verrall, Mrs. Fenwick, Mr. Cronshaw, Mr. Christian, Miss MacCallum, Miss Lloyd Still, Miss Peterkin and the Chairman.

It was decided to hold a further meeting of Council in a week's time to consider the rules regarding the Register, the Seal and existing nurses, and members were asked to send in resolutions for circulation.

Between May 11th and July 16th, six meetings were held in private and a large amount of business was conducted. It was resolved that the minimum age for admission to the Register was to be 21; that candidates must give evidence of good character from three responsible persons to cover the three years immediately preceding the application; that all persons (existing nurses) should before November 1st, 1919, have had one year's training in a general hospital or Poor Law Infirmary and two years subsequent practice; and that for existing nurses the

38

Registration fee should be 1 guinea with an annual retention fee of 2s. 6d.

There was much discussion on the Supplementary Registers and it was decided that there should be a Register of Fever Nurses and that the nurses of mental defectives should have a separate division in the Mental Nurses' Register. Details of the admission of existing nurses to the Supplementary Registers were discussed and it seemed obvious from the beginning that there might be some difficulties over mental nurses' registration.

It was further resolved that Standing Committees should be formed and that the Chairman was to be, ex-officio, member of all committees. Members were asked to say on which committees they wished to serve with the following results:

Registration Committee	Finance Committee	Education and Examination Committee	Disciplinary and Penal Committee
Mr. Christian	Mr. Christian	Miss Dowbiggin	Miss Cattell
Miss Coulton	Mr. Cronshaw	Mrs. Fenwick	Mr. Christian
Miss Cox-Davies	Miss Cox-Davies	Miss Lloyd Still	Mr. Cronshaw
Mrs. Fenwick	Mrs. Fenwick	Miss Sparshott	Mrs. Hills
Miss Dowbiggin	Miss MacCallum	Miss Swiss	Miss MacCallum
Dr. Goodall	Miss Lloyd Still	Miss Tuke or	Miss Macdonald
Miss Macdonald	Sir Jenner Verrall	Mrs. Hills	Miss Peterkin
Miss Peterkin	Miss Villiers	Miss Villiers	Sir Jenner Verrall
Chairman	Chairman	Miss Worsley	Chairman
		Chairman	

A special Standing Committee to consider the registration of mental nurses consisted of Mr. Christian, Miss Cox-Davies, Miss Dowbiggin, Dr. Goodall, Miss MacCallum, Dr. Bedford Pierce and Miss Lloyd Still.

Since it was obvious that the Council had no means of raising money until nurses started to register, and since it was equally obvious that they would have expenses, the Minister of Health offered to lend the Council £5,000. It is interesting to compare this figure with the balance sheet drawn up by Dr. Bedford Fenwick for the Select Committee in 1904 (see page 11).

There were four candidates interviewed for the post of Registrar: two conditions of appointment were given to them at interview, namely that the appointment was terminable by six months' notice on either side, and that the Registrar was to retire at the age of 60, with the Council having an option to extend this by two years. After interview, three successive ballots were held, eliminating the candidates with the lowest number of votes at each ballot. The candidate with the highest number of votes in every ballot was Miss M. S. Riddell.

Marian Scott Riddell was 48 at the time of her appointment; she had trained at St. Bartholomew's Hospital from 1901–4 and had then been a sister at her training school. In 1905 she went to University College Hospital as Night Superintendent and was appointed Assistant Matron there in 1908. In 1911 she went to the Chelsea Hospital for Women, as Matron, and on the outbreak of war she became Matron of the Second London General Hospital. In 1917 she was Matron of the Fifty Third General Hospital in France, and in 1919 went to the War Office as Acting Matron-in-Chief. She was offered the post of Registrar to the General Nursing Council and took up her appointment on January 24th, 1921.

All seemed to be going smoothly but in early July 1920 three questions were asked in the House of Commons. Mr. A. Davies asked the Minister of Health—was the Chairman (of the G.N.C.) appointed without consultation of members of Council, and if so, what was the Minister's authority for his action? Mr. R. Richardson asked—was the Minister aware that the Chairman had neither the experience nor knowledge of medical matters sufficient to enable him to understand and guide the General Nursing Council in its deliberations on professional subjects? Dr. Addison replied that he was under no obligation to consult the Council and there was no suggestion that it had been hampered in its work; he was aware "of foolish gossip which has nothing to do with the matter"[1]. It is impossible to know what led to these questions and they were only reported in one of the three nursing journals. However the Minister and Chairman of Council obviously took them seriously. At the sixth meeting of the General Nursing Council on July 16th, the Minister attended and the meeting opened with the Chairman reading the questions and stating that "he could not continue to occupy the Chair unless he felt he had the confidence of the Council". The Minister then addressed those present but what he said is not recorded! When he had finished, Lady Hobhouse moved "in view of the questions, recently asked in the House of Commons, this Council wish to disassociate themselves absolutely and entirely from such action and to express their deep regret that the capacity and efficiency of their Chairman should have been impugned thereby. They desire to express their great appreciation of his conduct of the business of the Council. In their judgement his impartial wisdom and skill have been used in the best interests and prestige of the important national work with which this Council has been charged." This was seconded by Sir Jenner Verrall and carried nem. con. The Minister then withdrew and the business proceeded. Perhaps it is significant that a resolution in Mr. Christian's name was passed that "the Council be open to the press, but that any member at any time could move that they went into camera". This was seconded by Miss Cattell and carried unanimously. The press were therefore present at the seventh meeting of Council, held on Friday, July 30th.

At this meeting the report of the special Mental Nurses Committee recommended that the certificate of the Medico-Psychological Association should be accepted by the Council for admission of existing nurses to the mental register during the period of grace. A resolution from the Education and Examinations Committee was carried, to the effect that nurses who produced a certificate of not less than three years' training from a general hospital or Poor Law Infirmary, which terminated at any period after November 1st, 1919, but before the Rules made by the Council for the education, examination and training of nurses became operative, should be admitted to the General part of the Register; similar provision was made for the supplementary registers, except for fever nurses for whom the standard then in force (two years' training and certification and one year's service) was agreed; these were to be the "intermediate" nurses.

After the holiday period, in August, when no meetings were held, the Council met monthly. One controversial question which was discussed was the registration of V.A.Ds. These were women who had nursed in military hospitals, for varying lengths of time, during the war, but who had received no formal training. There were many thousands of V.A.Ds. and nurses believed that if they were allowed to register, they would flood the labour market. The leaders of the profession, in all organisations, were determined to exclude them. The Council received a letter from the Central Joint V.A.D. Committee asking for a ruling on the State Registration of its nursing members, and after discussion a resolution was moved by Miss Cox-Davies that "the Central Joint V.A.D. Committee be informed that V.A.D. members who served in military hospitals are not eligible for registration". This was carried unanimously; the Chairman suggested that a letter be sent, containing the words, "we very much regret that our answer must be in the negative". According to one nursing journal this was met by a chorus, "No regrets"![2].

A slight hiatus arose over the discussion on the draft Rules; the Chairman of Council had ruled that this matter was sub-judice, but the *Nursing Times* published three columns on the subject with extensive comments—this produced a resolution at the October meeting that during the discussion of the Rules, the press be excluded. The Chairman pointed out that any member of Council could move that it should sit in camera; however, the resolution was seconded and carried unanimously and the rest of the meeting took place without the press!

Eighty-nine applications had been received for the post of Registrar's Assistant and Miss Parslowe was appointed in November—at about the same time Miss G. E. Davies was appointed Registration Clerk. By the end of the year the Finance Committee were able to report that a house, 12 York Gate, London, N.W. had been viewed and approved; staff were now being appointed and the offices had been found.

The year 1920 ended with the draft Rules still under discussion. Included in these had been provision for the Council to elect its own Chairman annually. The Minister of Health was not yet prepared to accept this and wished to keep the nomination in his own hands for the time being. A letter to the Council stated:

"The Minister recognises that when the Register has become securely established the Council may properly claim full discretion in the selection of its Chairman, but while he hopes that all nurses who are entitled to claim registration will avail themselves of their right, he cannot ignore the possibility that these hopes may not be realised and that the elected members of the second Council may be chosen by an electorate only partially representative of the profession: the Council are well aware too of the controversies which have divided the profession in the past, and while the Minister is confident that the Council will in the end be the means of securing unity, it would be unfortunate if the election of the next Chairman should become in any sense a trial of strength between more or less antagonistic sections. He therefore feels that, in the interests of the successful working of the Council . . . it is of the utmost importance that for the next four years the chairmanship of the Council should be held by someone whose impartiality and independence are beyond question, and on these grounds he would urge that the nomination of the Chairman should be left with him for the next four years and that any rule for the subsequent election of the Chairman by the Council should not come into force earlier than January 1925."

According to the minutes the Council felt unable to accept this, since they thought it wrong to commit the second, elected Council.

1921

By the beginning of 1921 the various committees were well established in their work.

TRAINING AND EXAMINATIONS

In November 1920 the Education and Examinations Committee, under the Chairmanship of Miss Lloyd Still, had drawn up a draft schedule for approval of training schools: this had been adopted by the Council. Six principles were laid down.

(1) There should be a "one portal" examination. This re-referred to a Preliminary examination which it was felt should be taken at the end of the first year by all nurses training for any of the Council's Registers. The object of this was to gain a remission in time for a nurse who chose to continue training to gain a second qualification.

(2) There should be a general standard of nursing education in all training schools.

(3) The principle of Preliminary Training Schools should be accepted. (At the time few hospitals had achieved this.)

(4) The term (or length) of training should be clearly prescribed.

(5) Hospitals were to be circulated with questionnaires, so that the Council could know the number of beds in each

institution, the clinical material available and other relevant details.

(6) There should be a minimum standard of general education for entry to nurse-training.

Early in 1921 Miss Riddell, at the direction of the Council, sent out the questionnaires to training schools; in addition to the points just mentioned, hospitals were asked to state the ratio of nurses to patients, the teaching staff available and the number of lectures given. This obviously took time and no lists of approved training schools were issued in 1921.

However in November the Committee, who had by now received replies to their questionnaires from most of the training schools, recommended that 50 beds should be the minimum number for an approved general hospital, with a daily average of not less than 35 occupied.

The main work of the Committee was concerned with the draft syllabuses for training and examination. This was to be one of the points at issue with both the Ministry and the training schools for the next four years. The Committee hoped that a syllabus of training, giving the content of lectures, would be approved by the Minister and would be compulsory for all training schools. By March 1921 a draft pamphlet of lectures and demonstrations for general training had been prepared and circulated to hospital and Poor Law Authorities and trained nurses' organisations; this was accompanied by explanatory notes, and invitations to an informal conference at the Royal Society of Medicine, to be held in April. The draft syllabus included a suggested "nurses chart" which was a record of practical work to be initialled by the ward sister. The draft and chart were largely based on the system of training devised by Miss Lloyd Still and Miss Gullan at St. Thomas's Hospital: the latter had the distinction of being the first appointed "Sister Tutor" in 1914.

The syllabus was divided into first year work and work in the second and third year of training.

The headings for the first year were:

(1) Anatomy and physiology.

(2) Elementary science including hygiene, sanitation and bacteriology.

(3) Theoretical and practical nursing.

44

(4) Food values and invalid cookery.

(5) First aid.

At the top of the page were the words "the submitted scheme is intended to be treated in the briefest outline. The amount of ground to be covered will show that the subject matter can only be touched on. Sections 1, 2, 4 and 5 and a brief outline of 3 can be included in a Preliminary School course, where such exists".

The headings for the second and third year were, anatomy, physiology, elementary science, gynaecology, surgery and medicine.

At the same time the Committee were considering the draft Rules for examinations. They suggested the subjects should be anatomy, physiology, elementary science (including hygiene, sanitation and bacteriology), first aid, gynaecology, materia medica, dietetics, surgical nursing and medical nursing. It was suggested that candidates must pass all subjects in the syllabus issued by the Council. Work was also going on on the syllabuses for the Supplementary Registers; the Mental Nurses Committee recommended that, for their training, the existing syllabus of the Medico-Psychological Association should be adopted for three years.

The Registrar's notice calling the conference on April 28th, on the proposed training syllabus stated that it "will be private and not open to the press, but as soon as possible after the meeting an official communication will be issued to the press for publication" The press comment on this was "Healthy differences . . . make for progress: the differences of view that are apparent in the Nursing Council are a healthy sign, and will do no harm as long as they can be threshed out publicly, so that the wider interests that are concerned may have clear ideas on the subject; but for some time there has been evident a disposition to deal with these matters behind closed doors . . . this secretive tendency appears to be thriving." The Editor's footnote to this comment from the Poor Law Officers' Journal agreed with it, but added that the Council had had a change of heart at the last moment and agreed to admit the press to the conference[3].

The conference, which was well attended, was opened by Mr. Priestley. There were three main speakers in the morning: Miss

Lloyd Still spoke on the draft syllabus, Miss Dowbiggin on "Aspects in relation to Poor Law Infirmaries" and Dr. Goodall on "The Medical aspects". This was followed by general discussion. Many of the audience agreed with Miss Musson, Matron of the General Hospital Birmingham, who felt happier after listening to Miss Lloyd Still, but still felt the draft syllabus was overcrowded. Some of the matrons of the smaller hospitals were concerned at the capabilities of their probationers to deal with the content of the syllabus. Others welcomed it and claimed that a Preliminary Training School was essential. The only two tutors whose comments were reported—one from The London and one from Lambeth Infirmary—both said the syllabus could work well.

Miss Cox-Davies summed up the morning session and reminded those present that the first year's work was only to be taught in the briefest outline.

In the afternoon the speakers were Miss Sparshott, Dr. Bedford Pierce and Miss Coulton, who read a paper for Miss Seymour Yapp, who was ill. The topics dealt with were reciprocal registration and the supplementary registers. Discussion again followed and Mrs. Fenwick summed up.

By the middle of the year it became obvious that many Poor Law Infirmary authorities were becoming gravely disturbed. Their attitude may be summed up by the following report, quoted in the *British Journal of Nursing*. The Hackney Guardians had received a recommendation from their committee to apply for approval as a training school and to adopt the curriculum laid down by the General Nursing Council. "We regret to note that Rev. A. H. Dacombe (why are the Clergy so reactionary?) said that if the Board adopted the recommendation it would put them under the coercive and tyrannical option of the General Nursing Council. Having alluded to the success of their present regime and the substantial cost that the appointment of a Sister Tutor would entail, he moved the reference back of the recommendation, which was supported and carried.

"We have no doubt wiser councils will prevail, as the Clerk pointed out that the running of the Infirmary was carried out economically owing to the large number of probationer nurses on the staff and in the event of the Infirmary not being recognised it would be difficult to attract probationer nurses, and that would eventually mean the employment of a highly paid staff of trained nurses"[4].

In July, the Council received a deputation from a conference of representatives of Poor Law Nurse Training Schools. Many of them were perturbed at their lack of candidates for training and at the poor education of those they had. Their spokesman thought that the first criticism met with of the syllabus of training was that it had aimed too high: however it was agreed that some Poor Law training schools had such a syllabus in operation and did not find it too difficult. "It looked terrible but was not as terrible as it looked!"[5]. The representatives asked that a syllabus of examination should take the place of the syllabus of training and also queried the need for Preliminary Training Schools in Poor Law Institutions. At the Council meeting which followed this deputation there was much discussion about the examination syllabus which was already being prepared: some members felt that it would be better to defer sending out the training syllabus until the examination syllabus was ready, but in the end it was agreed to adopt and publish the training syllabus at once and send a copy to the Minister for approval. Those in favour of the training syllabus included Mrs. Fenwick, Miss Lloyd Still, and Dr. Goodall, and those less happy included Miss Sparshott and Miss Worsley.

Progress continued on the training syllabuses for the fever and sick children's training and a letter was received from the Chairman of the Parliamentary Committee of the Medico-Psychological Association agreeing that a Preliminary Examination should be held for all types of hospital, which should be reciprocal. The Mental Nurses Committee decided to hold a conference of representatives of mental hospital training schools on the syllabus and schedule in November.

At the November Council meeting a letter was received from the Minister saying he was not yet prepared to accept the training syllabus, but wished to wait for the rules regarding examinations and affiliation of hospitals for training purposes.

As far as examinations were concerned the Education and Examinations Committee proposed that the first should be held in July and October 1923 and January and April 1924; these were to be voluntary. After April 1924 all nurses desiring to register must take the State Examinations; the first compulsory one was to be in July 1924, and then in January, April, July and October each year. At a later date, all nurses would have to take the Preliminary Examinations. Fourteen towns were chosen as examination centres and others were to be agreed later. The Final Examination was to cover two days and consist of two sessions of written papers and two sessions which included a viva and a practical.

THE SEAL, UNIFORM AND BADGE

Anyone reading The Nurses Rules Approval Instrument (1961) may be forgiven for being rather surprised to find that three and a half pages are taken up with minute detail of the official State Registered Uniform. Few S.R.N.'s today have ever seen this uniform and would certainly not be able to describe it. However in the Registration Act 1919 it is specifically stated that the Council "shall make Rules . . . with respect to the uniform or badge which may be worn by nurses so Registered", and it is obvious that the early Councils took this part of their work very seriously.

It was decided, in February 1921, that the Seal (which was to be used on every Registration Certificate) was to be a medallion with Hygeia (the goddess of health) in the centre, the rose of England on the right, the daffodil of Wales on the left, a scroll with A.D. 1919, and round the margin the title, "The General Nursing Council for England and Wales". It is interesting to note that the Scottish Seal incorporated the cross of St. Andrew and the Irish Medallion, a leaf of shamrock in each corner.

The question of the uniform and badge was thrown open to the profession who were asked to send in suggestions: one of the specific questions was whether the outdoor uniform should be a cloak and bonnet or a coat and hat. There was sufficient controversy for no details to be settled during 1921.

FINANCE, THE OFFICE AND THE STAFF

It will be remembered that the Council started its financial life with a loan of £5,000 from the Ministry of Health. In February 1921, the Finance Committee, under the Chairmanship of Sir Jenner Verrall, reported that the half yearly payments amounted to £684 11s. 7d. leaving a balance of £4,429 12s. 8d. The sub-Committee dealing with the house at

12 York Gate, London, N.W.1, were asked to keep expenditure on furniture etc. at about £1,500 and in the same month the signing of the lease was agreed. The house was handed over to the Council on March 17th; furniture was purchased up to £427 10s. 0d. and the decorating was estimated at £150. On June 10th the first headquarters of the General Nursing Council for England and Wales was opened by Her Royal Highness, Princess Christian. Mr. Priestley made an address of welcome and the Archdeacon of London invoked a blessing.

At the reception, Her Royal Highness had tea and members of Council, and others, were presented. Those present included the Mayor of St. Marylebone, Sir Arthur Stanley, Mr. Brock (Ministry of Health) and many of the distinguished nurses of the day. The house itself consisted of a basement and four floors; in the basement was a mess-room for clerical staff; on the ground floor a reception room, the Registration Department and the Assistant Registrar's Office; on the first floor the Committee Room and the Registrar's Office; on the second floor, offices and cloakrooms; and above, rooms for the housekeeper and her assistant.

In July 1921 the Finance Department announced the appointment of an Accountant, Miss Hatty Smith, and Council elected a General Purposes Committee to oversee the running of the office. This consisted of Mrs. Fenwick, Miss Cox-Davies, Miss Villiers, Miss Coulton and Miss MacCallum.

In November, the Finance Committee reported difficulties over the cost of advertisements in the nursing press. The *Nursing Mirror* had written to the Council saying that they would need to charge a higher rate than the flat rate being paid by the Council to all journals, of 7s. 6d. per inch. At the time the Registrar had been instructed to reply that if the flat rate were impossible, the advertisements could not be sent.

Now, Miss Sparshott proposed a resolution that "advertisements be inserted from time to time in all nursing papers, not withstanding their charge may not be the same", as she felt Council would wish their announcements to reach all nurses[6]. This provoked an argument: Miss Lloyd Still and Miss Cox-Davies agreed with Miss Sparshott but Dr. Hill, Miss MacCallum and Mrs. Fenwick were against. Mrs. Fenwick (still, at this time, the Editor of the *British Journal of Nursing*) specifically objected to the General Nursing Council being exploited by the *Nursing Mirror*, "for 30 years a rabid anti-registration organ"[7]. Finally an amended resolution was carried, that cost alone should not be a bar to the insertion of an advertisement in any paper.

In November too it was reported that three extra temporary clerical helpers were being employed at salaries of £2–£2 10s. per week. Replying to criticisms of the small salaries, Miss Villiers pointed out that there were now 13 clerical workers in the office and the annual expenditure on salaries was nearly £3,000. The increase in staff was mainly due to the fact that nurses were now beginning to register.

REGISTRATION

The main work of the Registration Committee, under the Chairmanship of Mrs. Fenwick, in the early part of 1921 was concerned with the Rules under which existing and intermediate nurses could register during the period of grace. One of the problems was that, because of reciprocity, the Minister insisted that the Rules should be similar for all three General Nursing Councils.

In Scotland there was difficulty over the fever nurses. The Scottish Board of Health, who for some years had held its own examinations, insisted that existing fever nurses should be placed on the General Register, whereas the English Council intended to place them on a Supplementary Register. The Board of Health submitted figures showing, that the number of fever nurses on their register was 1,137 of whom 622 had had further general training; allowing for death, marriage, etc. they felt it seemed probable that only a small number of existing fever nurses without any general training would want to register[8].

From March to June considerable feeling was aroused over this, questions were asked in the House of Commons and representatives of the three General Nursing Councils met to discuss the matter and details of the fees.

On July 7th a deputation went to the Minister composed of representatives of the Royal British Nurses' Association, the Matrons' Council, the Registered Nurses' Parliamentary Council, The National Union of Trained Nurses, the Fever Nurses' Association, the College of Nursing Ltd., and the Pro-

Second Schedule.

FORM I (a).

THE GENERAL NURSING COUNCIL FOR ENGLAND AND WALES.

Nurses' Registration Act, 1919.

Application for Registration for Existing Nurses for Admission to the General Part of the Register.

To the General Nursing Council for England and Wales.

1. Full Christian names and Surname. (1) I, *Ethel Gordon Fenwick*

2. Place and date of birth. (2) *Spynie House, nr Elgin, Morayshire. N.B.*
   January 26th 1857

3. State here whether single, married or widow. If married or widow, give maiden name. (3) *Married. Ethel Gordon Manson.*

4. Full Postal Permanent Address. (4) ~~*20 Upper Wimpole St. London W.1.*~~
   Rt: form 25/9/24. 12, Barton Street, Deans Yard,
   Westminster, S.W.1.

hereby request the General Nursing Council for England and Wales to enter my name upon the General Part of the Register of Trained Nurses maintained by the Council.

I forward herewith the fee of One Guinea*, and I promise, in the event of my being so registered, and in consideration thereof, to be bound by, and to conform in all respects to, the Rules and Regulations for the time being in force.

5. If no certificate is held explain the reason.

(5) I forward herewith my Certificate of Training (and copy of the same) from *Certificates were not awarded to Paying Probationers at Nottingham & Manchester.*

The following are the places in which and dates of the times during which I was *bona fide* engaged as a nurse in attendance on the sick:—

PLACES.	DATES.			
	Month	Year	Month	Year
The Children's Hospital, Nottingham, Paying Probationer.	From *1st April*	*1878*	to *September*	*1878*
Royal Infirmary, Manchester Paying Probationer.	From *Sept 1878*		to *Sept*	*1879.*
London Hospital. 2 Sisters.	From *Sept 1879*		to *April*	*1881.*
St Bartholomew's Hospital. E.C. Matron & Supt of Nursing.	From *May 1881*		to *August*	*1887.*

A.&E.W.—82022.

T.O.

(a)

3. An 'existing nurse's' application for registration:
   (a) front   (b) back

50]

I hereby declare that the above particulars are in every respect complete and true.

Signature of Applicant _Ethel Gordon Fenwick_

Signature of Witness _Margaret Breay_

Address of Witness _431 Oxford St London W.1._

One of such persons shall be a householder, not being a relative of the applicant, who has known her personally for not less than three years, and the others shall be persons, such as matrons of hospitals, registered medical practitioners, or other responsible persons under whom the applicant has worked.

Date _September 2⁴, 1921._

Name and Address of Referee as to Character.

_Miss Henrietta Hawkins. P.L.G.
124. Friern Barnet Road
New Southgate_

Names and Address of Referees as to Character and Professional efficiency.

(1) _Miss Margaret Breay
431. Oxford St.
London. W. 1._

(2)

* If a nurse's application for registration is not accepted the Guinea Fee will be returned.

3. (b).

fessional Union of Trained Nurses. The deputation stated that "much unrest was felt at the delay in publishing the Rules for the admission of existing nurses. They took the greatest exception to admitting Scottish fever nurses to the Scottish General Register and so by inference to the English Register."

The Minister of Health—now Sir Alfred Mond—said that the Secretary of State for Scotland had now agreed to withdraw this proposal and he (Sir Alfred) was ready to sign the Rules, subject to the reciprocity rule being deferred.

At an emergency meeting of the General Nursing Council on July 14th it was agreed unanimously to defer the reciprocity rule and the Minister signed the Rules the same day. Editorial comment in one of the nursing journals on announcing the fact, said that this date was "an auspicious augury to students of French history"![9]

Announcement of the Rules were made in the press and existing nurses urged to obtain application forms from the Registrar and to forward them on completion together with the appropriate fee and documents.

Arrangements were made for the Registration Committee to scrutinise the applications and to submit recommended names to Council. The first Register was to be published in July 1922.

The Rules stated that all nurses who completed three years general training or one year's training and two years' service before November 1st, 1919 might be registered as existing nurses in the general part of the Register, if approved by Council, during a two-years' term of grace from July 14th, 1921 on payment of a fee of 1 guinea.

From, and after, November 1st, 1919, nurses must hold a certificate of three-years' training from a general hospital or infirmary approved by the Council, and might be registered as intermediate nurses on the general part of the Register, if approved by the Council, upon the payment of a fee of 2 guineas. The general part of the Register was reserved for female nurses whose legal title was "Registered Nurse". The Register contained supplementary parts for the registration of male nurses, mental nurses, sick children's nurses and fever nurses both for existing and intermediate nurses.

Readers should compare the Rules with the wording of the Act, particularly as it refers to bona fide nurses. The Rules were signed by the Minister of Health and lay before the House of Commons for the statutory 21 days before becoming law. During this period no member of Parliament, nor of the nursing profession, raised any query.

Mrs. Fenwick, in triumph, set off to tour the country to explain the Rules to the nurses. Also, in her capacity as Chairman of the Registered Nurses' Parliamentary Council, she wrote to Sir Alfred Mond and Dr. Addison to thank them.

During August the Council had its summer recess but the journals were full of information on why, how and where to Register. September came full of high hopes, but peace was soon to be shattered.

In September a special committee for classifying applications met three times a week, to prepare papers for the Registration Committee as many applications were being received. According to her own memories, Mrs. Fenwick scrutinised every application personally. One problem, which was highlighted in the press, arose over the registration fee: when the College of Nursing opened its own register, before the 1919 Act, a promise had been made that no further fee would be required when the State Register was opened. However, since the College Bill did not become law this could not happen and College members found themselves paying a second fee. After considerable discussion in the press the College agreed to refund 1 guinea to anyone applying for it.

At the General Nursing Council meeting on September 30th it was announced that 1,816 applications for registration had been received (£1,912 3s. 11d. in fees), of these, 366 nurses were recommended for the general register,

14 nurses for the fever register

1 nurse for the mental register.

It is of interest to note, that in the general register:

No. 1 is Fenwick, Ethel Gordon (née Manson)

	Tr. 1878–1879
No. 2 is Lloyd-Still, Alicia Frances Jane	Tr. 1896–1899
No. 3 is Cox-Davies, Rachael Annie	Cert. 1893–1896
No. 4 is Sparshott, Margaret Elwin	Cert. 1892–1895
No. 5 is Dowbiggin, Annie	Cert. 1896–1899
No. 6 is Yapp, Charlotte Seymour	Cert. 1900–1903

No. 1 in the fever register is Bryant, Annie   Exp. 1894–1896
No. 1 in the mental register is Christian, Tom
                                    Cert. M.P.A. 1900–1903
By October the nursing press was commenting on the value of the hospital certificate of training. There had obviously been discussion as to whether it was necessary for the original document to be sent to the Council when applying for registration, but (said the *British Journal of Nursing*) "how else can the Register be accurate?"[10].

Another point about hospital certificates was highlighted at the October Council meeting. Miss Cox-Davies, who had been ill and had missed earlier meetings, proposed in a resolution that the word "certificated" in the Register should be reserved for those who would later be admitted by virtue of examination, and that all existing and intermediate nurses should simply be entered as "trained". Miss Cox-Davies did not like dividing existing nurses into trained and certificated and pointed out that "one large hospital had in the past given only one and two years certificates and some gave evidence of training in the shape of writing". Miss Dowbiggin seconded this and quoted St. Thomas's as giving no certificates between 1877–1904.

Mrs. Fenwick was annoyed and voluble—first this matter should have been referred to the Registration Committee and not the Council; and second "the resolution contained an unprecedented proposal of a most disastrous nature calculated to wreck the Register". Nurses, she added, would have a real grievance if their hard earned certificates were not recorded— no Medical or Nursing register had ever been compiled, depriving (she would not use the word defrauding) the persons admitted of their professional qualifications; she would stump the country to prevent injustice being done[11]. It will be noted that Mrs. Fenwick's entry in the Register does not contain the word "certificate"—so she was not fighting for herself.

The Chairman said Mrs. Fenwick was threatening the Council and that the word certificate was not mentioned in the first Schedule, which laid down what was to be entered in the Register.

Mrs. Fenwick pointed out that the insertion was provided for in the Rules.

The argument continued for some time: Miss Cox-Davies

was backed by the Chairman, Miss Lloyd-Still and Miss Dow-biggin, and Mrs. Fenwick by Miss Villiers, Mr. Christian, Miss MacCallum and Dr. Goodall. Finally Miss Cox-Davies with-drew her resolution.

Letters about the inclusion of the word "certificate" appeared in the nursing press on both sides and finally Mr. Brock, from the Ministry of Health wrote to say that the Council could not vary the particulars set out in the first Schedule without sub-mitting an amended Schedule which must receive the Minister's sanction.

At the November Council meeting Mr. Brock's letter was read, and also many from nurses, objecting to their certificates not appearing in the Register.

Mrs. Fenwick gave the report of the Registration Committee which included details of a heated argument about the certifi-cates with the names of those who voted for and against; those for the inclusion of certificates were Mrs. Fenwick, Mr. Christian and Miss Macdonald; those against, Miss Cox-Davies, Miss Dowbiggin, Miss Peterkin and Dr. Goodall.

One member of the Registration Committee objected, in Council, to part of the report and the Chairman of Council ruled that it should be struck out of the minutes. However, Mrs. Fenwick strongly objected to "the mutilation of the report"[12] and subsequently published it in its entirety in the *British Journal of Nursing*. At this point the Council went into camera and there is no further record of what happened.

THE END OF 1921

By this time, the Chairman obviously felt he could not con-tinue: he was sensitive to public criticism and twice before in July 1920 and in April 1921 had threatened to resign over questions in the House of Commons. On December 10th the *Nursing Times* reported that he and two thirds of the General Nursing Council had tendered their resignations to the Minister —but not, it was stated, over the question of the certificates. In the same edition there was a letter from Lord Knutsford which included the comments that Registration was useless, that few had applied and that the fee was too high; his advice to nurses was "wait and see". He was answered the following week by "Matron" who said that Registration was useful, that Lord

Knutsford had been a life-long opponent, that nurses wanted a State Register and should register at once.

In the *British Journal of Nursing*, Mrs. Fenwick described the resignations as a "strike". On the date on which the December Council meeting should have been held, five members attended, Mrs. Fenwick, Miss Villiers, Miss Macdonald, Miss MacCallum and Mr. Christian. Apologies for absence were received from Miss Dowbiggin and Miss Cattell. The members waited 15 minutes and as there were not enough to form a quorum, they adjourned.

On December 21st, Mr. Brock saw the members who had resigned, and later stated, "the resignations had nothing to do with the question of the syllabus or the entry of certificates of qualification of existing nurses in the Register"[13].

References

1. *Nursing Times*—17.7.20.
2. Ibid—2.10.20.
3. Ibid—30.4.21.
4. *British Journal of Nursing*—9.7.21.
5. Ibid—16.7.21.
6. Ibid—5.11.21.
7. Ibid.
8. Ibid—March 1921.
9. Ibid—23.7.21.
10. Ibid—21.10.21.
11. Ibid—5.11.21.
12. Ibid—26.11.21.
13. *Nursing Times*—31.12.21.

Chapter 4

THE CARETAKER COUNCIL (2)

"From committees, charity and schism: from philanthropy
and all the works of the devil, Good Lord deliver us."

FLORENCE NIGHTINGALE

For the first weeks of the new year (1922), the profession could only speculate on the future of the General Nursing Council. Throughout January the Minister stated that he was not yet in a position to make an official pronouncement about the resignations: the press comment was, "presumably the trouble has not yet been adjusted. We sincerely hope the members will withdraw their resignations: indeed we do not doubt that their loyalty to the nursing profession will lead them to do so, provided of course, that they will have some guarantee that the present difficulties will not arise again"[1].

It is obvious that there was much activity behind the scenes, and equally obvious that a great deal of it concerned Mrs. Fenwick; she herself recorded that she was seen at the Ministry and asked to resign as Chairman of the Registration Committee —this she refused to do[2]. Whether because of this or not, Mr. Priestley would not withdraw his resignation, and in early February his successor was appointed.

Major-General Sir Wilmot Herringham, K.C.M.G., C.B., M.D., F.R.C.P., became the second Chairman of the General Nursing Council: he was a consultant physician at St. Bartholomew's Hospital, and according to a provincial newspaper "showed courage in accepting the appointment on a body whose brief life has not been a very harmonious one"[3]. It is interesting to note that he and Mrs. Fenwick were old acquaintances: as well as being connected with the same hospital, they had grown up in the same village. Mrs. Fenwick remembered that "when I was three years old my widowed mother married Mr. George Storer, Lord of the Manor of Hawkesworth . . . Sir Wilmot Herringham's father was at that date Rector of Hawkesworth"[4]. It would appear that they had not been particularly friendly even as children!

The other members of Council withdrew their resignations, but it was clear at the first meeting of 1922 that certain specific

56

changes had been agreed with the Minister. This meeting took place on February 3rd and all business was accomplished in the record time of 75 minutes. Two notices of motion were announced, both designed to alter and speed up the process of Registration. Dr. Goodall proposed a motion "to enable Council to accept, in place of a nurses' hospital certificate, a duly certified copy of such a certificate, or a declaration on the part of a responsible official of a nurses' society or association that a certificate had been produced to that body". Miss Cox-Davies said she would move that it be an instruction to the Registration Committee to examine only those cases submitted for registration which appeared doubtful, and to delegate the routine work to the Registrar.

At the next meeting, on February 17th, these motions were debated. Dr. Goodall pointed out that it was essential to get as large a number of Registered nurses as possible by September 30th, when the election procedure had to start. Applications were coming in at the rate of 700 a month, but approvals were far fewer. Sir Jenner Verrall drew a parallel with the first Registers for doctors and dentists when all those in bona fide practice were registered without question. After much discussion the resolution about certificates was approved by 15 votes to 6—this division of votes and viewpoints corresponded to the split at the end of 1921. The same divergence of opinion was to be seen throughout the whole of 1922.

When Miss Cox-Davies' resolution was debated Mrs. Fenwick again repeated that so far she had personally scrutinised every single application: she objected to "an official being given power to say who should or should not be registered: it was establishing a bureaucracy in the office"[5]. On being put to the vote the resolution was carried by 16 to 6.

Towards the end of the meeting the majority group in the Council showed its strongest weapon. Miss Coulton moved an alteration to the Rules, "that each Committee appointed in 1920 and 1921 should go out of office on the date of the first ordinary meeting after the Rule came into operation, and new Committees be appointed by Council at that meeting. Thereafter the said Committees shall be appointed annually at the first Ordinary Meeting each January"[6]. She said that there were some members who had never served on a committee and it was right to give every member a chance of doing so. Mrs. Fenwick pointed out forcibly that this would result in the minority group not being placed on certain committees again. The Chairman's reply was surprisingly curt as he must have known that this was exactly what was going to happen: "the rules of debate are the rules of good manners and the rules of good manners are not to impute to those with whom you are arguing opinions other than those they profess, especially not feelings of personal antagonism or enmity"[7]. The resolution was agreed by 16 to 6 and a meeting called for February 24th (in one week's time) to put the Rule into effect. It is obvious that Sir Wilmot had reason to anticipate the Rule being signed immediately but, on this occasion, he forgot the power of Parliamentary procedure and Mrs. Fenwick's influence. No meeting was held on February 24th but questions were asked in the House of Commons. Mr. Alfred Davies asked the Minister if he had promised to sanction this Rule before the General Nursing Council had met on February 17th, and if not, how had the Chairman known that sanction was assured? Two other members suggested that the representatives of working nurses were being penalised, by the power of matrons and employers of nurses on the Council. The Minister said "the Chairman had consulted me and I am prepared to sanction Rules to speed up registration. The Council consider that a reconstruction of existing committees will expedite the formation of the Register and the experience of the last six months leads me to share their view"[8].

The Rule was signed and at the Council Meeting on March 17th the committees were re-appointed: Mrs. Fenwick and Miss Macdonald both lost their seats on the Registration Committee, and Dr. Goodall was elected its new Chairman. Letters of protest were received from the Professional Union of Trained Nurses, the Registered Nurses' Parliamentary Council and the Royal British Nurses' Association. The six "minority" members wrote declining to accept office on any Standing Committee from which one or more "minority" member had been excluded. As these were accepted and covered most of the committees, Mrs. Fenwick's group found itself with only the full Council as its debating ground.

On March 23rd, in the House of Commons, Major Barnett

put forward a motion to annul the new Rules but this was defeated by 64–49. The Minister's reply summarised the position: he pointed out that this "was an old squabble" and the result of a feud between two different nursing associations— one championed by Major Barnett. He had only managed to get the Council members to withdraw their resignations by promising to support them. He said that out of 50,000 nurses, 3,235 had applied to become Registered and only 984 had been accepted; it was vital to have a speeding up of machinery, since in eight months time Registered nurses had to elect a new Council. If the new Rules were rejected he would have no other course open to him but to repeal the Act and do away with the Register altogether[9].

The "old squabble" had been followed with interest and concern in the press and all must have agreed with the *Lancet*'s comment—"we hope the work of reconstruction will be allowed to proceed"[10].

Once the committees had been re-appointed the main work of the Council continued.

EDUCATION AND EXAMINATIONS

Since the Minister was unwilling to sign the training syllabus, the Education and Examinations Committee decided to speed up the drafting of the examinations syllabus and to call a conference with representatives of the Poor Law Infirmaries and others to discuss this. It seemed likely, in view of the delay, that the examination dates would have to be deferred. The conference was held at the Robert Barnes Hall in Wimpole Street; it was emphasised that the syllabus of examination must be based on the syllabus of training. Most of those present and especially the Guardians of the Poor Law Hospitals were far happier with the examination syllabus, and a spirit of co-operation rather than criticism was evident. The difference in the two syllabuses lay in the fact that the new one listed subjects on which candidates might be examined, whereas the previous one had specified lecture material to be covered at different points in training. In August, the Association of Poor Law Unions wrote to the Minister of Health: they were happier about the examination syllabus, but the training syllabus still troubled them; they felt that it required a standard of general education far in advance of many of their candidates, especially with regard to the scientific subjects. Following this, the Minister wrote to the Council saying that he was not prepared to do anything about the training syllabus until he had the examination syllabus before him.

After much discussion the Education Committee agreed to recommend that the syllabus of examination and the "nurses' chart" should be published together. The examination was to be in two halves—Preliminary and Final: the 1924 examination was to be voluntary, for any existing nurses who had not registered and the compulsory examinations would start with the Preliminary in 1924 and the Final in 1925. It was suggested that the training syllabus should be advisory and not compulsory. This last point caused considerable controversy in the ensuing Council meeting, and Mrs. Fenwick was voluble about the fact that only one nurse had been present at the meeting of the Education Committee which had "scrapped the syllabus".

During the year, the first lists of approved training schools were published: in March, 111 voluntary hospitals were approved—the London list beginning with Charing Cross and ending with the West London—a total of 22, and the provincial list of 89, beginning with Ashton-under-Lyne District Hospital and ending with York County. In June, 62 Poor Law Hospitals were approved, 25 in London beginning with Bermondsey and Rotherhithe and ending with Willesden Infirmary, and 37 in the provinces, beginning Lake Hospital, Ashton-under-Lyne and ending with New Cross Infirmary, Wolverhampton. At every Council meeting for several years these lists continued to be published and to this day changes in approval appear in the minutes of each meeting.

The published Rules for approval included such points as the number of beds—for a voluntary hospital, 100, with a daily average occupancy of 75, and for a Poor Law Infirmary, 250: that there must be at least one resident medical practitioner: and that experience must include medicine, surgery, gynaecology and children's diseases. Special rules were made for grouping of hospitals unable to fulfil these conditions and for affiliated training. The Education Committee also considered that adequate staff and equipment for teaching should be provided and that Preliminary Training Schools should be set up in various centres in England and Wales.

Specific rules were made for training schools for the supplementary registers.

Some of these proposals provoked much comment and the Poor Law Association again wrote to the Minister pointing out that 25 of their hospitals would be excluded as training schools through not having a resident medical officer. Any regulations were obviously going to cause hardship to someone, and from the outset the Council was faced with the problem, which still pertains today, of maintaining similar standards in a large number of hospitals with differing facilities and service demands.

FINANCE

During the early months of 1922 the slow progress of registration caused some anxiety to the Finance Committee since expenditure threatened to overtake income. However, with the increased number of successful applications the position improved and the audited accounts for June showed that the Council had met the necessary expenditure and still showed a balance. By August £2,500 of the original loan from the Ministry had been repaid and in September, having £6,753 in hand, Council agreed to free itself from debt and repay the rest. In November £3,000 was invested in War Loan and the Committee were much happier about the general position.

THE OFFICE AND STAFF

Until the signing of the Rules in June 1921 and the opening of the Register, the work of the office staff was not heavy. However, once nurses began to apply, the amount of sorting, checking and writing for references increased each month, until by the middle of 1922 the staff were having to work on Sundays to keep pace with it. Added to this, the staff and particularly the Registrar became more and more involved in the arguments between the two factions on the Council. At one meeting, members were arguing so violently about procedure and efficiency in the office, that the *Nursing Times* reporter was quite unable to hear what was going on for several moments[11].

The General Purposes Committee had already looked at the

work of the office, but following criticism the Chairman personally inspected this. In his report he stated "the work presses hardly on the head of the registration room. She is responsible for the work of the whole room: she conducts all correspondence and personally checks the finer details of the work. But it presses most hardly of all upon the Registrar, who is responsible for all work and has to spend much time in preparation for and attendance on meetings and in addition has to see a large number of people. It is, I think physically impossible for her to carry out all the work that requires to be done just now." As a result of this, extra assistance was recommended and later in the year a Registrar's secretary was appointed.

In the autumn, with the forthcoming election in mind, the Minister agreed to the temporary employment of additional clerks.

The effect of all the controversy was hardest on Miss Riddell, and in September, she asked for an outside expert inspection of the whole office work: this was eventually agreed. In November, not surprisingly, she became ill and was away for several weeks.

REGISTRATION

The progress of registration continued to be stormy. In February the question of the use of the word "certificate" in the Register was settled by Miss Cox-Davies withdrawing her resolution and Mrs. Fenwick moving an amendment to the First Schedule, on the form of the Register, which was carried.

In March, once the new Rules had been passed and the Registration Committee re-appointed, a letter was received from the executive committee of the League of the Royal Free Hospital Nurses asking that the League might be recognised by the Council in accordance with the new rule. It will be remembered that Dr. Goodall had proposed that a declaration by an official of a responsible nurses' association that a certificate had been seen, should obviate the need to send in original certificates. The Registration Committee recommended to Council that this should be accepted. This request was followed by a similar one from the College of Nursing Ltd., which provoked lengthy arguments but was finally agreed 12–6. The "minority" group were opposed both to the Rule and the College!

By now the Registrar was dealing with all straightforward applications and only referring doubtful ones to the Registration Committee. At the time of the re-organisation of committees, four doubtful applications had been placed in a drawer by Mrs. Fenwick to await a new rule on conjoint training. Miss Riddell had honestly believed that all applications in the drawer had been passed as being in order and had let these through. They had been formally approved by Council in April but before names had been entered in the Register or the applicants informed, the next crisis arose, as Mrs. Fenwick called at the Council's offices and happened to find the relevant papers. As the leader in the *Nursing Times* stated in a slightly desperate tone, a resolution was put down for the next Council meeting in Mrs. Fenwick's name "that as four of the 20 applications, passed as eligible by the Council on April 21st, and since scrutinised, have been found not to conform to the Statutory Rules, the instruction to the Registration Committee . . . granting discretion to the Registrar be rescinded . . . and the Council be saved the risk of litigation"[12].

The problem of the four nurses and this resolution, provoked bitter discussion which brought up all the old enmities and attracted much comment from the press.

In June the Registration Committee, to whom the problem had been referred suggested to Council that as the applicants had not been informed, the Registrar be instructed not to enter their names in the Register. Mrs. Fenwick immediately pointed out (quite correctly) that this was not in order since as Council had passed the names, only Council could remove them. The whole problem dragged on for months.

Despite all this, applications were being dealt with much more quickly: all those registered by the September Council meeting were eligible to vote in the ensuing election. By July this came to 6,616 out of a total of 8,516 applications.

The number of applications aroused some comment: it was natural to wonder why so few had applied out of a potential electorate of 50,000, and a known College membership of 20,000. There was also comment by Mrs. Fenwick and Miss MacCallum on the 6,616, since they maintained that the Register was being "packed" and preferential treatment given to College members and nurses from the Royal Free. In view of this it is interesting to look at an analysis of the first 500 names on the Register—all of which had been approved by Mrs. Fenwick herself. The 500 names represented trainees of 214 hospitals including the 12 London teaching hospitals.

136 training schools showed 1 Registered nurse
42　,,　,,　,,　2　,,　nurses
15　,,　,,　,,　3　,,　,,
6　,,　,,　,,　4　,,　,,
3　,,　,,　,,　5　,,　,,
5　,,　,,　,,　6　,,　,,
2　,,　,,　,,　7　,,　,,
3　,,　,,　,,　8　,,　,,

Of the London teaching hospitals the numbers were:

University College Hospital	2
Westminster Hospital	3
St. George's and King's College Hospitals	5 each
Royal Free, St. Mary's and Charing Cross Hospitals	6 each
The London Hospital	7
Middlesex Hospital	10
St. Thomas's Hospital	12
Guy's Hospital	13
The Royal Hospital of St. Bartholomew	53

The 6,616 names appeared in the first published Register, but the actual electorate by the time voting papers were issued was over 12,000.

Reciprocity

One of the problems which faced the Council was the question of reciprocal registration not only with Scotland and Ireland but also with other countries, in the (then) Dominions and Crown Colonies. This involved detailed scrutiny of their training programmes to see whether they were sufficiently similar to allow a foreign trained nurse to be registered in England and Wales. Winston Churchill, then Secretary of State gave advice over the question of the Crown Colonies and at that time (1922) saw no point in negotiating with any except British Guiana, Jamaica and Trinidad. Other problems in such countries as Canada and Australia were due to the fact that individual states or provinces had their own training arrangements and registration laws. One of the earliest countries with whom reciprocal arrangements was made was New Zealand. This aspect of the Council's work continued to increase over the years. In 1949 the Council's powers were widened and they were able to accept for registration suitably trained nurses from any country.

THE ELECTION

The 1919 Registration Act stated that the first election was to be held "in accordance with the prescribed scheme and in the prescribed manner": the prescription was drawn up by the Registration Committee, before its re-organisation and according to Mrs. Fenwick had followed as closely as possible the principles adopted by the Minister in nominating the Caretaker Council. The Committee suggested that the following should be elected:

(a) 6 past or present matrons of training schools for nurses to be elected by those on the general register.
   (i) 4 of general hospitals—one at least provincial.
   (ii) 2 of Poor Law Infirmaries—one provincial.
(b) 5 registered nurses (not matrons) one of whom must be in the public health service, to be elected by those on the general register.
(c) 1 fever nurse ⎫
(d) 1 sick children's nurse ⎪ each to be
(e) 1 male nurse ⎬ elected by
(f) 2 mental nurses—one male, one female ⎪ those on the
                        ⎭ supplementary registers

The election was to be held by ballot and voting papers were to be sent out by post; each nurse was to have one vote for each place in the class in which she was registered. In discussion, many of the nurse members of Council were against dual voting but the recommendation was finally passed.

When the Minister received the scheme he wrote about the specific seats for matrons. Subsequent alterations resulted in an equal division of matrons' seats between the metropolitan areas and the provinces, and the inclusion of a private nurse in the five seats for registered nurses. Candidates for election had to be nominated by six of their colleagues.

At a special meeting in October the election procedure was decided. Neither the Returning Officer, nor his deputy were to be nurse-members of Council. Twenty-one days before the election, a notice was to be published in two or more newspapers circulating in England and Wales, Scotland and Ireland; the form of the notice was specified. Details of nomination papers were laid down and if the nominated persons "do not exceed the number to be elected, such persons shall be deemed to be elected". Voting papers were to be sent out seven days at least before the last day fixed for their return.

At this stage the College of Nursing Ltd. arranged a meeting to choose candidates whom they would support. This support was bound to influence the election since no other organisation had the facilities, or money to support an election campaign; their nominees were obviously only for the matrons and general registration seats since at this time only female general trained nurses were elegible for College membership. Fourteen nominations were put forward. The Minister introduced a further complication by laying down that a nurse who had at some point been a matron of a small hospital might stand as a candidate in the non-matron category. At this point, as things were getting very complicated, Mrs. Fenwick asked if the whole election could not be thrown open and no specific seats allocated: this was not put to the vote.

The "minority" group who described themselves as independent candidates, held several meetings. The journals each published their lists of favoured candidates. Fourteen independent nominees were put forward, and three candidates were unopposed—Miss Seymour Yapp, Mr. Stratton and Miss Villiers.

Once the election procedure was under way it seemed that the Caretaker Council's troubles were over. However, one last mischance had to be overcome. Sir Wilmot Herringham, in his capacity as Returning Officer, had attempted to please the minority group who insisted that the Council's staff should not be involved in the election, by employing an outside firm. The latter sent some nurses two voting papers instead of one and over 1,000 nurses received none at all. The *Nursing Times* commented "it will be seen that the first General Nursing Council has surpassed itself and added a crowning error to its record.

CANDIDATES STANDING FOR ELECTION TO THE GENERAL NURSING COUNCIL.

A	Miss R. COX-DAVIES, R.R.C.	Matron, Royal Free Hospital, London.
	Miss E. LLOYD STILL, C.B.E., R.R.C.	Matron, St. Thomas' Hospital, London.
	Mrs. BEDFORD FENWICK	Past Matron, St. Bartholomew's Hospital, London.
	Miss HEATHER BIGG, R.R.C... ...	Past Matron, Charing Cross Hospital, London.
B	Miss M. E. SPARSHOTT, C.B.E., R.R.C.	Matron, Royal Infirmary, Manchester.
	Miss E. M. MUSSON, R.R.C.	Matron, General Hospital, Birmingham.
	Miss C. ALCOCK, R.R.C.	Past Matron, Royal Hospital, Portsmouth.
	Miss H. L. PEARSE	Past Matron, North Staffordshire Infirmary; present Superintendent of Nurses, L.C.C.
C	Miss ALSOP	Matron, Kensington Infirmary.
	Miss J. F. BALLANTYNE, A.R.R.C. ...	Matron, Fulham Infirmary, Hammersmith.
D	Miss C. SEYMOUR YAPP ...	Matron, Lake Hospital, Ashton-under-Lyne.

E	Miss MABEL ANSLOW ...	Registered Nurse,	Matron's Assistant, London Hospital.
	Miss DOROTHY S. COODE ...	Ditto,	Head Preliminary School, St. Thomas' Hospital.
	Miss GERTRUDE COWLIN ...	Ditto,	Librarian, College of Nursing.
	Miss FLORENCE M. EMBREY	Ditto,	Matron, Swithland Home, Loughborough.
	Mrs. M. I. STEWART WATSON	Ditto,	Proprietor Nursing Home, Sheffield.
	Miss VIOLET JANE WEBSTER	Ditto,	Superintendent School Nurses, Leeds.
	Miss DOROTHY WINDLEY ...	Ditto,	Sister Tutor, Paddington Hospital.
	Miss MAUDE MacCALLUM ...	Ditto,	Hon. Secretary, Professional Union of Trained Nurses.
	Miss ISABEL MACDONALD ...	Ditto,	Secretary, Royal British Nurses' Association.
	Miss GERALDINE BREMNER	Private Nurse.	
	Miss E. A. CATTELL	Ditto.	
	Miss S. M. MARSTERS	District Nurse, (Supt. Marylebone-Paddington D.N.A.).	
	Miss ELLINOR SMITH	Ditto, (Q.V.J.I. Supt., Wales).	
	Miss E. C. SWISS	Public Health Nurse (formerly Health Visitor, Willesden)	
	Miss C. C. du SAUTOY	Public Health Nurse (formerly Q.V.J.I. Inspector, Wales)	
	Miss E. WADE	Public Health Nurse (	

F	Miss A. M. COULTON	Matron, East London Hospital, Shadwell (Children's).
	Miss A. M. BUSHBY	Matron, Queen's Hospital for Children.
G	Miss S. A. VILLIERS	Matron, South-Western Fever Hospital.
H	Mr. FREDERICK WM. STRATTON ...	Trained Male Nurse, Hackney Union Infirmary.
I	Mr. TOM CHRISTIAN	Chief Charge Nurse, Banstead Mental Hospital.
	Mr. ROBERT DONALDSON	Manager, Male Nurses' Co-operation and Mental Nurses' Association, Hinde Street.
J	Miss H. M. PERRY	Matron, Cardiff City Mental Hospital.
	Miss M. E. WIESE	Chief Charge Nurse, Claybury Mental Hospital.

NOTES ON THE VOTING.

(1) *Votes of Nurses on the General Register.*

A. These are four matrons (past and present) of London General Hospitals, of whom nurses may vote for *two* only.

B. Four matrons (past or present), of Provincial General Hospitals, of whom nurses may vote for *two* only.

C. Two London Poor Law matrons, of whom nurses may vote for *one* only.

D. One Provincial Poor Law matron, unopposed, for whom one vote may be cast.

E. Sixteen Registered nurses, of whom only *five* may be voted for in all, *but* three of these votes should be given in Section E1 (Registered nurses), one in Section E2 (Private nurses), and one in Section E3 (Public Health and District nurses).

(2) *Votes of Nurses on the Children's Nurses' Register.*

F. Two matrons of Children's Hospital, of whom nurses must vote for *one*.

(3) *Votes of Nurses on the Fever Register.*

G. One matron of a Fever Hospital (unopposed) for whom one vote may be given.

(4) *Votes of Nurses on the Male Nurses' Register.*

H. One general-trained male nurse (unopposed), for whom one vote may be given.

(5) *Votes of Nurses on the Mental Nurses' Register (Male).*

I. Two male mental nurses, whom nurses may vote for *one* only.

(6) *Votes of Nurses on the Mental Nurses' Register (Female).*

J. One matron and one charge nurse, of Mental Hospitals, of whom nurses may vote for *one* only.

4. Candidates standing for the first election (1922).

GENERAL NURSING COUNCIL
ELECTION.

The most *IMPORTANT NOTICE*
TO
STATE REGISTERED NURSES
IS TO
VOTE

When you have read your Voting Paper very carefully, put your cross opposite the following names:—

General Part of the Register.

Two Matrons from Metropolitan Hospitals.
Miss A. F. J. **LLOYD STILL**, C.B.E., R.R.C., Matron of St. Thomas's Hospital, S.E.
Miss R. A. **COX-DAVIES**, R.R.C., Matron of the Royal Free Hospital, W.C.

Two Matrons from Provincial Hospitals.
Miss E. M. **MUSSON**, R.C.C., Matron, General Hospital, Birmingham.
Miss M. E. **SPARSHOTT**, C.B.E., R.R.C., Matron, Royal Infirmary, Manchester.

One Matron Metropolitan Poor Law Hospital.
Miss H. A. **ALSOP**, Matron of Kensington Infirmary.

One Matron Provincial Poor Law Hospital.
Miss C. **SEYMOUR YAPP**, Matron, Poor Law Infirmary, Ashton-under-Lyne.

Five Registered Nurses.
Representing District Nursing—
Miss E. **SMITH**, Superintendent, Q.V.J.I.N., Chester.

Representing Private Nursing—
Miss G. **BREMNER**, Private Nurse, Nurses' Co-Operation, Langham Street, W.1.

Three other Nurses—
Miss D. S **COODE**, Sister Tutor, Preliminary Training School, St. Thomas's Hospital, S.E.

Miss G. **COWLIN**, In Charge of Library and Information Bureau, The College of Nursing, Ltd.

Miss E. C. **SWISS**, formerly Public Health Nurse, Willesden Borough Council.

Supplementary Parts of Register.

1 Registered Male Nurse.
1 Registered Mental Nurse (Male).
1 Registered Mental Nurse (Female).
Miss H. M. **PERRY**, Matron, Whitchurch Mental Hospital, Cardiff.
1 Registered Sick Children's Nurse.
Miss A. M. **COULTON**, Matron, Shadwell Hospital, E.
1 Registered Fever Nurse.
Miss S. A. **VILLIERS**, Matron, South-Western Fever Hospital, Stockwell.

Present Member of the General Nursing Council.

5. The College of Nursing candidates, 1922.

ADDRESS OF INDEPENDENT CANDIDATES

TO THE

ELECTORS OF THE GENERAL NURSING COUNCIL FOR ENGLAND AND WALES.

The Independent Candidates must apologise for again addressing the constituency of the Nurses' Direct Representatives on the General Nursing Council for England and Wales. In doing so, those of their number who were members of the Council whose term of office expired on December 23rd, 1922, disclaim any responsibility for the breakdown in the system and method of the Election, as the Council was not consulted in regard to the details by the Returning Officer, who assumed and acknowledges entire responsibility for placing the clerical work in the hands of persons not responsible to the Council.

NAMES OF CANDIDATES.

The Independent Candidates who offer themselves for election to represent Registered Nurses on the General Nursing Council are :—

General Part of the Register.

MRS. BEDFORD FENWICK.
MISS MILDRED HEATHER-BIGG, R.R.C.
MISS HELEN L. PEARSE.
MISS JESSIE F. BALLANTYNE, A.R.R.C.

MISS SUSAN M. MARSTERS.
MISS ALICE CATTELL.
MISS ISABEL MACDONALD.
MISS MAUDE MacCALLUM.

MISS CATHLIN CICELY DU SAUTOY.

Supplementary Parts of the Register.

MISS ALICE M. BUSHBY - - - Sick Children's Nurses.
MR. TOM CHRISTIAN - - - - - Male Mental Nurses.
MISS MAUD E. WIESE - - - - Female Mental Nurses.

(Two Independent Candidates, Miss S. A. Villiers (Fever Nurses) and Mr. F. W. Stratton (Male Nurses) have been declared elected without a contest.)

The majority of the above Candidates are well known to the Electorate.

As their Election Address has already been submitted for your consideration, together with the portraits of the majority, they hope it is unnecessary to send you second copies.

PROFESSIONAL POLICY.

The Independent Candidates desire, however, once more to bring to your notice the professional policy for which they stand, because the efficiency of educational standards, the value of State Registration to Nurses and the public, and the financial stability of the General Nursing Council for England and Wales largely depend on the knowledge, courage, and ideals of the persons elected to form the forthcoming General Nursing Council.

They stand firmly for the Statutory Rights incorporated in the Nurses' Registration Act, 1919, few of which Registered Nurses at present enjoy owing to the reactionary policy, and lack of sympathy with nursing ideals, of the majority of the members of the First Council.

6. The independent candidates, 1922.

Reg: No.	Name (if Married, Maiden Name)	Permanent Address	Date of Registration	Qualifications
1	Fenwick (née Manson) Ethel Gordon	20, Upper Wimpole Street London. W1.	30.9.1921	Royal Infirmary Manchester Trained 1878 & 1879
2	Still Alicia Frances Jane Lloyd	St. Thomas' Hosp¹. S.E. 1	30.9.1921	St. Thomas' Hospital. London Trained 1896 – 1899
3	Cox-Davies Rachel Annie	2 Greville Street, Brunswick Square, London W.C.1. Royal Free Hospital Grays Inn Rd W.C.1.—	30.9.1921	St. Bartholomew's Hospital & c. Cert 1895 – 1896
4	Sparshott Margaret Elwin	Royal Infirmary Manchester.	30.9.1921	General Hospital Nottingham Cert 1892 – 1895
5	Dowbiggin Annie	North Middlesex Hospital Edmonton. N.18.	30.9.1921	General Infirmary Leeds Cert 1896 – 1899
6	Deceased April 1934 Yapp Charlotte Seymour	Fabre Hospital Mellor Road Ashton-under-Lyne. Lancs.	30.9.1921	Aston Union Infirmary Erdington Birmingham Cert 1900 – 1905
7	Villiers Susan Alice	South Western Hospital Landor Road S W 9.	30.9.1921	St. Bartholomew's Hospital. London Cert 1892 – 1895

7. The first page of the manuscript Register.

[67

If the election is null, owing to an error, surely the whole election is invalid: we imagine that nomination papers must be signed afresh and new nominations accepted"[12]. However, all previous nominations were allowed to stand and new voting papers were issued. Questions were asked in the House of Commons about irregularities in election procedure, but members were assured that these were covered in the 5th schedule of the Representation of the People Act 1918. The Chairman's explanation was that the whole thing was a sheer mistake, but this in no way calmed those members who thought a grave injustice had been done; it was decided that the new ballot papers should be issued by January 10th, 1923 and returned by January 24th. The 30th and final meeting of the Caretaker Council, on December 15th, lasted three and a quarter hours and was held in an atmosphere of mistrust and anger. As laid down by Parliament, the first Council was dissolved within three years of the passing of the Registration Act, without its successors being known.

One is apt to remember the publicity of the squabbles, and enmities; in fact one should bear in mind the tremendous amount of work achieved, which laid the foundations of all the future work of the Council.

References

1. *Nursing Times*—14.1.22.
2. *British Journal of Nursing*—22.12.23.
3. *Nursing Times*—4.2.22.
4. *British Journal of Nursing*—22.12.23.
5. *Nursing Times*—25.2.22.
6. Ibid.
7. Ibid.
8. Ibid.—4.3.22.
9. Ibid.—1.4.22.
10. Ibid.
11. Ibid.—27.5.22.
12. Ibid.—20.5.22.
13. Ibid.—9.12.22.

Chapter 5

THE FIRST ELECTED COUNCIL, 1923–1927

"It is a common aphorism that people are governed as they deserve."
ETHEL G. FENWICK

The election results were announced at the end of January, and were as follows:

General hospital matrons:

Miss R. A. Cox-Davies	5,179 votes	London
Miss A. Lloyd Still	5,169 „	
Miss E. M. Musson	5,378 „	Provinces
Miss M. E. Sparshott	5,531 „	

Poor Law hospital matrons:

Miss H. A. Alsop	4,614 votes	London
Miss C. Seymour Yapp	Unopposed	Provinces

Registered nurses:

Miss E. Smith	3,786 votes	Public Health nurse
Miss G. Bremner	4,064 „	Private nurse
Miss D. S. Coode	3,372 „	
Miss G. Cowlin	3,094 „	
Miss C. C. du Sautoy	2,711 „	

Male nurses:

Mr. F. W. Stratton	Unopposed

Mental nurses:

Miss M. E. Wiese	294 votes
Mr. R. Donaldson	265 „

Sick Children's nurses

Miss A. M. Bushby	102 votes

Fever nurses:

Miss S. Villiers	Unopposed

The appointed members were:

By the *Privy Council*:
Lady Hobhouse
The Hon. Mrs. N. L. Hills

By the *Board of Education*:
Miss A. S. Barrett
Sir Wilmot Herringham

By the *Ministry of Health*:
Rev. G. B. Cronshaw
Dr. E. W. Goodall
Dr. Bedford Pierce
Dr. Smedley
Sir T. Jenner Verrall

The press comments were interesting. The *Nursing Times* stated, "and if we may presume to offer advice to the new members, we would suggest that they all take a course of lessons in the conduct of meetings and in the Rules laid down by the Act so that they may be sure of their ground"[1]. The *British Journal of Nursing* launched a bitter attack on the whole election procedure and pointed out that "where the electorates for the supplementary candidates could not be influenced (Rule 9a) by the College—as the general part of the Register has been—every vacancy has been filled by an independent candidate! the rest of the elected members of the Council are nominees of the College of Nursing Ltd., the majority of whom are members of its Council"[2].

It must be remembered that Mrs. Fenwick was still editor of this journal and had just lost her seat: but as so often in her writing, her facts remained accurate, however "coloured" her attitude.

The new Council met on February 16th; despite the fact that the offices had been established at York Gate for some time, there was no room big enough for the full Council and these meetings were still being held at the Ministry.

The meeting began with the announcement that only one person had been nominated as Chairman—and Sir Wilmot Herringham then took the Chair; he had received seven nominations, five of them from elected nurses. He told the Council that most of its work—especially the detail—was done by committees, but that major policy must be decided by the Council itself; he reviewed the work of each committee, said that he had no doubt that the Council had not any idea of the immense volume of work, and added that that of the Education and Examinations Committee was likely to be the hardest. One new member had obviously already decided to devote a large part of her time to the Council's work, since in February Miss E. M. Musson resigned from her post of Matron of Birmingham General Hospital. The returning officer's statement about the election gave the following facts. The electorate on January 10th, 1923 was 12,097 of whom 10,887 were on the general Register, 24 on the male part, 639 on the mental part, 191 on the sick children's part and 356 on the fever part. 11,495 voting papers were issued, of which 8,715 were returned. The cost of the election was £635 9s. 1d., and the second ballot had cost £116 18s. 0½d.

At this same meeting a further 1,505 names were approved for Registration. Accusations were made, in a letter to Council that 800 of these "were non-College members whose applications had been delayed as the officers refrained from sending out reference papers in time". This letter, from Miss Mac-Callum, a copy of which was sent to the Minister, stated that the Register had been "packed" in the interests of the College. Council asked to be informed of the exact number who had in fact been Registered under Rule 9a (by which an officer of a responsible body, could verify possession of a hospital certificate), and were told that of the 12,097 electorate, 1,243 were passed as College members, six as members of the Royal Free Hospital Nurses' League, and 824 by barristers, J.P.s, etc. Questions about the election were also asked in the House of Commons.

At this first meeting, the report by an outside firm—Messrs. W. B. Peat & Co.—on the work of the office was received. It covered 27 pages and was subsequently published by the Council. It confirmed that the Registrar and her staff were very overworked and that some work was in arrears because, until recently, the staff had been too small; in the circumstances, the organisation as a whole was good and no radical changes were suggested. It was difficult to make recommendations on future staffing, owing to the problem of assessing the future work of the office.

The new Council, with its five-year term of office, had five months in which to complete the registration of existing nurses; had to undertake the registration of intermediate nurses; and had to agree finally on the syllabus on which the future examinations would be run.

BONA FIDE NURSES AND THE CHAPPLE AMENDMENT

At the Council meeting in June 1922, one year after the Rules had been signed, the Chairman announced that a letter had been received from a Miss Herbert, of Porchester Square, London. She pointed out the unfairness of the Rules admitting existing nurses to the Register: the Act stated that during the period of grace, bona fide nurses could register if they had been engaged in practice as nurses for at least three years before November 1919; the Rules, however, went beyond this and said that they must have done a year's training and Miss Herbert contended that the Act did not justify this. Sir Wilmot considered the letter sufficiently important to be referred to the Registration Committee, with power to ask the Minister for advice. The *Nursing Times*, rather belatedly, said it had always been worried about this matter.

In March 1923, a letter was received from the College on the same point: it asked that existing nurses should be considered "on their merits, rather than on rigid rules". The Minister (now Mr. Neville Chamberlain) also wrote commenting on the inelasticity of the present Rules. It was generally felt, however, that at this late stage it was inequitable to make any substantial alteration unless this was endorsed by the bulk of the profession: there was obvious fear that if one year's training was abandoned, this might let in the V.A.D.'s. A strong argument at the time was the fact that registration was not compulsory for employment as a nurse and so no unfairness was created. However, Council were prepared to change the Rule for nurses who could "satisfy by length of practice". Rule 9(1)g was drawn up stating that any nurse who was in practice before 1900 and was still practising on November 1st, 1919 should be eligible for registration. The Scottish Council had agreed to this two years previously, and it would effectively keep out the V.A.D.'s.

In April Miss Herbert wrote to the *Nursing Times*. She pointed out firstly that, in practice, there was no distinction between the trained and untrained nurse, and before 1919 there had been no standard as a guide. Secondly that although non-registered nurses could still practice, it was likely to become more difficult;

and thirdly that because the General Nursing Council had no compulsory powers, it should be "diplomatic and statesman-like"; leaving a large group out would create a second standard, and it should be made possible for as many as could to register[3].

At the end of April the Parliamentary Medical Committee wrote to the *British Medical Journal*. Its spokesman, Dr. Chapple, suggested a new framework of Rules under which existing nurses could register: its main points were that any bona fide nurse of good character, who produced (1) a certificate stating that she had been in practice for a period of three years before November 1919, signed by a matron of a general hospital and two medical men; and (2) a second certificate signed by three medical men, saying that she had adequate knowledge and experience of medical and surgical nursing and was competent, should be eligible to register provided that, if necessary, she passed an examination set by the Council. He also asked for a Select Committee to enquire into the functioning of the Registration Act.

On May 11th, a special committee of the General Nursing Council met to discuss the letter and found they could not agree with the suggestions. The *Nursing Times* editorial, that week (after pointing out that only two months were left of the period of grace), quoted a letter from Sir Wilmot to the *British Medical Journal* stating that Dr. Chapple's proposal was retrograde and the Council "stuck to 1900". The *Lancet* agreed with Dr. Chapple[4].

The College had become involved on both sides: while welcoming Rule 9(1)g, some of its members had also had discussions with the medical Parliamentarians.

In early June, the 1900 Rule, 9(1)g, was before the House of Commons for approval: two amendments were put down—one of them being Dr. Chapple's.

The House heard all the previous arguments, and in addition Dr. Chapple stated that the College agreed with him. Major Barnett was opposed to the amendment and so, up to a point, was the Minister. Mr. Chamberlain said that the Act did not exclude the unregistered from practising, as had the midwives and dentists' Acts: he wanted the voting to be on party lines but was eventually forced to agree to a free vote: on this, Dr. Chapple's amendment was passed.

At the General Nursing Council meeting on June 15th the Chairman announced that the House had agreed to a motion praying the King, in Council, to modify the General Nursing Council's existing Rule. The Order in Council would probably be made before the end of the month, which would leave some two weeks before the end of the period of grace. In fact the King signed the Order on July 7th.

The General Nursing Council and all professional nursing organisations deplored the Chapple amendment. A statement issued by the Registration Committee and endorsed by the Council, stated that consideration should have been shown to those who *had* registered and that it should not have been left to the eleventh hour to alter so completely the character of the Register. Sir Arthut Stanley wrote to Dr. Chapple objecting to the statement that the College Council was in favour of the amendment, when in fact it was opposed[5]. The National Council of Trained Nurses, the Royal British Nurses' Association and the Registered Nurses' Parliamentary Council all presented petitions to the King in Council "against the admission of untrained persons" to the Register[6]. The Association of Hospital Matrons' Executive "viewed the new development with alarm," since it would depreciate the value of the State Register. The Poor Law Matrons' Association conveyed "very great regret", and the Secretary of the College of Nursing Ltd., sent a copy of a resolution passed at the Annual Meeting "deeply regretting that the House of Commons had decided to petition His Majesty to supersede the statutory duty of the General Nursing Council"[7].

Dr. Chapple maintained that he was right in spite of all criticism, and the comment of one historian on these events was that they were a triumph of Parliamentary democracy[8].

The fact is that the Act had not been interpreted strictly, but the original Rule had been drawn up in good faith by the Council, signed by the Minister and laid before Parliament in July 1921; no comment was made at that time.

In 1923 everyone realised the need to modify the Rule for existing nurses, but only non-nurses wished for as drastic a change as the Chapple amendment. As only seven days were left, further negotiation was impossible.

The Council realised that further protests were a waste of

time and concentrated on the flood of applications for Registration. Dr. Chapple attempted to get the period of grace extended since he maintained that the two years should start on the date the new Rule was signed: however, he was unsuccessful. In 1924 the Minister (Mr. Wheatley) informed him that he did not wish to pursue that matter any further, since the Council had no power to extend the date and he saw no necessity for consulting the Law Officers of the Crown.

During the last six months of the period of grace for existing nurses, applications were as follows:

1923	January	1,583
	February	1,706
	March	2,240
	April	2,328
	May	3,425
	June	6,273
	July (1st–14th)	4,345

This made a total of 21,900. The total number of existing nurses applications was 40,436, and of these 1,157 applied under Rule 9(1)g.

REGISTRATION 1923–7

Once the registration of existing nurses was complete, the "intermediate" nurses began to register: these were those nurses who completed three years training after November 1st, 1919, in an approved training school, but before the Council's examinations came into force in 1925. Their "period of grace" ended on June 30th, 1925.

The figures for the last few months were as follows:

1925	January	440
	February	610
	March	738
	April	904
	May	1,660
	June	4,852

The total number of applications for intermediate registration was 13,137.

Each year the Register was published and each year, in the

Council minutes, long columns of names appeared of those who had failed to pay their annual retention fee and so could not be included. Every nurse was sent two reminders, and to illustrate the work that was involved one can quote the following figures as examples: in the month of June 1924, 800 names were removed for non-payment, and in January 1926, 2,069.

As at this time, one-quarter of the Council's income was derived from these half-crowns, this also affected the financial position.

By 1927 reciprocal registration arrangements had been established with the Irish Free State and most of the States of Australia.

EXAMINATIONS

Early in 1923 a letter was received from the Minister, agreeing to the new examination dates. Following this, details were discussed and decided. The entry fees suggested were £2 2s. for the Preliminary Examination and £3 3s. for the Final Examination, with re-entry at half these fees. The Chairman of the Finance Committee, supported by Sir Wilmot Herringham, pointed out that the examinations must pay for themselves and that each part of the Council's offices must be self-supporting. However, some members—particularly Miss Wiese—felt that such fees quite exhorbitant and that many nurses, especially those in the mental field, would not pay them. After much discussion the fees were agreed.

Both examinations were to be held quarterly, if required, in July, October, January and April of each year; the written part could be taken at any centre where there were more than 25 candidates, provided a room and an invigilator were available. Fourteen centres were chosen for the practical part and it was decided that each nurse must bring her schedule or chart to the practical examination.

To enter for the Preliminary Examination, candidates must have completed one year's training; to enter for the Final Examination, candidates must have passed the Preliminary Examination, must have completed the prescribed training and have attained the age of 21 years. Prospective candidates had to apply not more than twelve weeks and not less than nine weeks before the examination; each candidate had to pass in all parts and would be notified individually of the results. The whole pass list would be issued in alphabetical order. Successful candidates would be sent a certificate, and the name would be entered in the appropriate part of the Register.

The actual content of the examination was to be as follows: for the Preliminary Examination there were to be two papers of $1\frac{1}{2}$ hours each, a 20-minute oral and a 30-minute practical. The Part 1 paper was to be in anatomy and physiology, three questions had to be answered, one in anatomy, one in physiology and the third in either. The Part 2 paper was in nursing and hygiene—three questions had to be answered, one of which must be hygiene and one nursing. The oral and practical examinations were to include all subjects.

The Final Examination was to consist of one paper of $1\frac{1}{2}$ hours in medicine, surgery and gynaecology, one paper of $2\frac{1}{2}$ hours in medical, surgical and general nursing, a 20-minute oral and a 30-minute practical.

Once the details had been agreed the Council had to find a panel of examiners. These were to be appointed twice a year, and were to be eligible for re-appointment, but as a rule should not serve for more than four consecutive examinations. Once the examinations were underway, it was realised that these last suggestions were quite impracticable. The Board of Examiners to set the papers were to be chosen from the panel, and from the outset the Council stated that all examiners were to be jointly and severally responsible for every question contained in the papers and the copyright was to be vested in the Council; these last still apply. The fees and subsistence allowances to be paid to examiners were also decided.

Obviously at this time relationships between the Council and the press were improving since after the meeting when all these details were announced a comment was "we welcome whole-heartedly what we hope is a change of attitude to the press. The courtesy of the Chairman, who repeatedly inquired as to whether the press had this or that document, was marked. We can hope for the continuance of this practice"[9].

Early in 1924, a sub-committee was set up to scrutinise applications for membership of the panel of examiners, and by April the first Boards were announced. Since the Preliminary

Examination was the first to be held, this was the first listed; its members were:

The Hon. Gertrude Best, S.R.N. (Assistant Matron St. Thomas's Hospital)

Dr. J. A. Nixon, F.R.C.P. (Bristol General Infirmary)

Dr. H. W. Jones, L.R.C.P., F.R.C.S. (Liverpool)

Miss Woodward, S.R.N. (Matron, Halifax Infirmary)

1,787 candidates entered for the first Preliminary Examination in June 1924, and 123 for the optional Final Examination. Many of the candidates must have been grateful for articles on "how to meet examination problems" which appeared in the press and a story illustrating these must have found an echo in the hearts of many: "A little girl at her prayers was heard to say 'Please, dear Lord, make Albany the capital of the State of New Jersey'. 'Why, Mary,' said her mother, 'that's a very strange prayer; why do you want God to to that?' 'Because,' said Mary, 'that's the way I made it in my examination this morning' "[10].

The results of the first Preliminary Examination were: 1,526 passed, 201 failed. Of the 201, 70 failed anatomy and physiology, 49 failed hygiene and nursing, 34 failed the oral, 79 failed the practical, and 3 candidates were below the average. It was remarked that several candidates failed in more than one subject, and many read the instructions incorrectly. At the following Council meeting the Chairman remarked that "the plough was only one of 11·4 per cent, which was very small and very satisfactory".

The *Poor Law Officers' Journal* pointed out that 650 of the candidates (2 out of 5) were trained in Poor Law Hospitals . . . and several voluntary hospitals, including The London, sent in no candidates at all, for this, the first of the great State Examinations[11].

By the time the second examination was complete, complaints began to be received about the wording of some questions. Miss Lloyd Still (Chairman of the Education and Examinations Committee) pointed out that it was very difficult to set a question simply, and implied that the Boards needed time to settle down. Some comments were made that questions had been asked outside the syllabus; all were passed to the Boards, or relevant oral or practical examiners.

In 1925 it was decided that the examinations should be held three, not four times a year. During the year comments continued in the press on hospitals who did, or did not, enter candidates for the State Examinations and their successes or failures. It was perhaps because of this that, at the end of the year, the Council decided not to publish details of the failures in future. The only London voluntary general hospitals to enter nurses for the first compulsory Final Examination were Prince of Wales Hospital, Tottenham, and Queen Mary's Hospital; they entered four between them, and all passed. The London Poor Law Hospitals had 95 candidates and 89 passed. The total was 395 entered of whom 326 passed.

By 1927 the State Examinations were well established. Inevitably comments began to appear in the press that nurses were becoming too examination minded. "Can she nurse her cases, was the question asked once, not has she passed her examination. And now the converse position has been created for since the General Nursing Council brought the examination test into the profession, as a permanent element, the difficulty has been to adjust so practical a profession to the exigencies of theoretical tests . . . the public are apt to judge the efficiency of a training school by the number of successful candidates"[12].

An interesting suggestion made during the lifetime of this Council was that there should be a higher examination for matrons. However, nothing came of this!

THE SYLLABUS

During 1923 the new Council accepted that the syllabus of training should only be advisory, and Mr. Neville Chamberlain agreed to sign the Rule making the examination syllabus compulsory. In February 1925 Mr. Wheatley signed the syllabus for mental and mental deficiency nursing. Later in the same year, in response to requests for more detail from examiners, explanatory notes on the examination syllabus were published. The *Nursing Times* commented: "the Council has been the victim of circumstances; both the Poor Law Authorities and the Ministry of Health pressed it to do what it did not want to do, namely, to substitute the syllabus of examination for the syllabus of training. To this it unwillingly consented, persuading itself that the former was but an abridged version of the latter. Lately, however, we find the State examiners condemning the syllabus as unworkable"[13].

The Education and Examinations Committee later revised the syllabus and this was signed by the Minister at the end of 1925.

MENTAL NURSES

It will be remembered that for many years the Royal* Medico-Psychological Association had organised its own training and examination for mental nurses. In the early days of the Council the Mental Nurses Committee had adopted the Royal Medico-Psychological Association training syllabus and had recommended that the examination should be recognised for registration of mental nurses during the period of grace. At the end of 1923 the Minister pointed out that it was undesirable to have two bodies examining for the mental Register. However, the Council was determined that mental nurses should be on the same footing as their colleagues and should take the same Preliminary Examination and a similar Final Examination. Several meetings took place in 1924 between members of Council and of the Royal Medico-Psychological Association, and in April 1925 it was announced that from June the Council would no longer recognise the Royal Medico-Psychological Association certificate for the purposes of registration. However, the Association announced that it would continue to hold its own examination. Two female mental nurses were particularly vocal at this time: Miss Wiese, as a Council member, fought hard for a reduction in mental nurses' fees for examinations, and attempted on every conceivable occasion to obtain special concessions for them; at more than one Council meeting she came into headlong collision with other members and Sir Wilmot Herringham, for trying to do what she felt to be her duty by a minority group. On the other hand Miss Macaulay, Matron of Kent County Mental Hospital, worked outside the Council to uphold everything it was trying to do to make mental nurses' training, examinations and registration exactly equivalent to that of their general colleagues.

UNIFORM

At the first meeting of the new Council, Sir Wilmot said that he felt that, as the people most interested, all the elected nurses

* The Medico-Psychological Association had received a Royal Charter in 1925.

should be members of the Uniform Committee! This was agreed.

By May they had completed and approved unanimously the details of the official uniform, badge, and registered letters over which the first committee had done so much work; the uniform was to be as follows:

(1) *Coat*—long coat, or coat and skirt. Skirt to be not less than eight inches and not more than twelve inches from the ground: or coat-frock with small detachable cape for outdoor wear. The material to be of two weights, and navy-blue in colour: for summer wear, showerproof gabardine; for winter wear, serge. Buttons—bone, with Tudor Rose in the centre and the lettering "England and Wales" round. Braid—artificial silk braid, $\frac{3}{4}$ inch wide in all, $\frac{1}{8}$ inch either edge in navy and centre $\frac{5}{8}$ inch royal blue.

(2) *Hat*—for winter wear, velour (blue). For summer wear, straw (blue). Trimming—navy blue ribbon with woven badge similar to badge chosen. Storm cap—of same material as coat, with braiding on flat, and woven badge in front.

(3) *Shoes*—black or tan. Stockings—black or tan or grey.

(4) *Gloves*—tan, grey or white.

(5) *Shirt* (to wear with coat and skirt)—white silk or cotton with polo collar fitting up to the neck.

(6) *Tie*—blue Irish poplin (same colour as centre of braiding).

The committee recommended that the badge submitted by Messrs. Fattorini, of Birmingham be adopted. The name, registration number and date of registration were to be engraved on the back. The badge itself, in blue and silver, had the General Nursing Council monogram in the centre and the words England and Wales round it. The same firm still make the badges today.

It had been decided, in 1922, to ask the Admiralty for permission to use the letters "R.N." as the official abbreviation of "Registered Nurse". However, this proposal was not acceptable to the Lords Commissioners of the Admiralty and in 1923 the following abbreviations were decided: S.R.N. (State Registered Nurse), R.M.N. (Registered Mental Nurse), R.N.M.D. (Registered Nurse of Mental Defectives), R.S.C.N. (Registered Sick Children's Nurse), and R.F.N. (Registered Fever Nurse).

The badges were duly registered at the patent office. Nurses

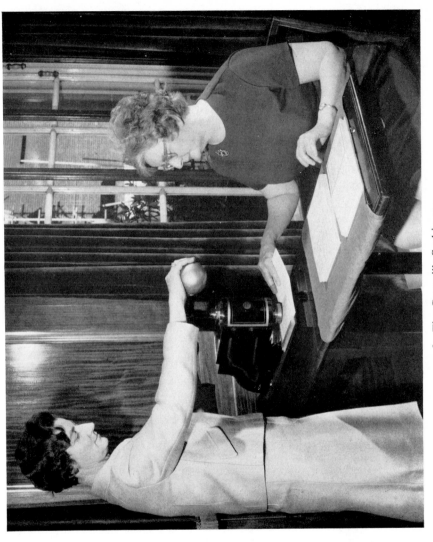

8. The Council's Seal in use.

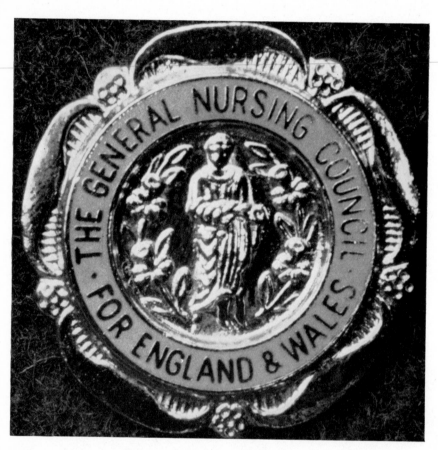

9. The State badge.

were waiting—many eagerly—for a chance to wear the registered uniform but the Minister delayed signing the necessary Rules until the early autumn of 1924. Tailors and outfitters had to apply to the Council for permission to make the official uniform which remained popular, particularly in London and the Home Counties until the 1939 war. A member of the Council's staff remembers the first day that the Registrar and Assistant Registrar appeared proudly at the offices in their uniform.

Every month, minutes of the Council meeting gave the names of several new official suppliers and over the years minor changes in style were made to keep the uniform up to date. To obtain the uniform, registered nurses required a permit from the Council's offices and in the period under discussion over 1,000 of these were issued each year. Today, every newly registered nurse receives a uniform permit with her Registration Certificate. Uniform has always been a "talking point" amongst nurses, and in the early days of the registered uniform it was a source of pride to many—but obviously not to all! The Editorial Notes in the *Nursing Times* read, "we still see many unsightly uniforms worn by registered nurses. The uniform, as designed, can look smart, but it is curious how few nurses succeed in looking smart in it. We should like to ask the State Registered Nurse we saw last week, who was wearing brown shoes with latticed laces half way up the leg, to discontinue this fantastic mode, which is an infringement of the regulations. But for the speed of the bus in which we were travelling we should have enlightened her personally"[14].

DISCIPLINE

One of the Council's important functions is the investigation of any complaint brought to its notice by individuals or by the Courts, which concern registered nurses and to institute proceedings against those who falsely represent themselves as being registered. In the Act, the General Nursing Council was empowered to make Rules concerning discipline and it also laid down the ways in which an individual so disciplined could appeal. A Disciplinary and Penal Committee had been in existence since 1921.

In 1924, it received a letter from the executive committee of the Chief Constables' Association for the Cities and Boroughs of England and Wales, asking for advice and possible action "against persons who improperly wear the dress of a nurse as a cloak for offences against the law". The first disciplinary action took place in September of the same year, when the Head Constable of Reigate notified the Council that a registered nurse had been convicted of a felony and sentenced to six months in prison. Against the wishes of some members, the case was heard in camera, but the sentence was announced in public and the Registrar was directed to remove the nurse's name from the Register.

THE STAFF AND OFFICES

During the years 1923–7 the work of the office staff changed considerably. During 1923 they had to cope with the flood of existing nurses who applied to register—and these at times reached 1,000 a week. From then on, first the applications from intermediate nurses and then the collection of annual retention fees and the compiling of the Register each year occupied the Registration Department. In 1924 the Examinations Department came into being and its work increased steadily. Additions to the senior staff included the appointment of an Examinations Officer, Miss Mackirdy, and a book-keeper to assist the Accountant. In 1924 Miss Parsloe resigned as Assistant Registrar and 38 applications were received for her post. Miss G. E. Davies—who had resigned from being Registration Clerk the year before—was appointed.

In 1926 the Minister approved a new recommendation on staff salaries and at that time the total salary bill was £7,338 per annum; with the new scales this rose to £9,114 per annum. By the end of 1927 the Council's staff numbered:

> Registrar's department—6
> Education and Examinations department—13
> Registration department—17
> Finance department—5
> Uniform department—2
> Postal department—3

At the Council meeting in December 1923, 12 York Gate was discussed: the house was already proving inadequate for the work and moreover it was only held on a short lease. In

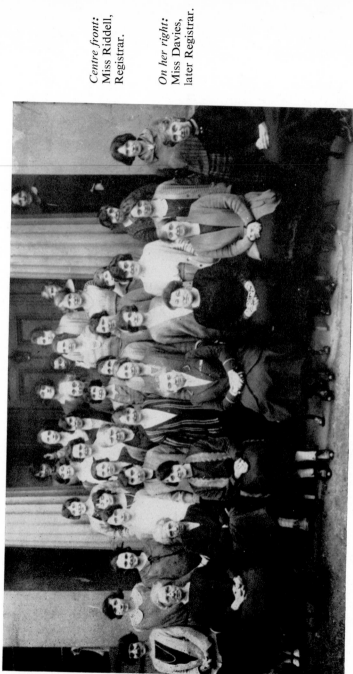

Centre front:
Miss Riddell,
Registrar.

On her right:
Miss Davies,
later Registrar.

10. The Council's staff in 1925.

January 1924 there was a report of preliminary negotiations to buy 20 Portland Place, London, W.1—a much larger house. It was described as being "beautiful premises, in a comparatively quiet street and was available for £5,500". The Finance Committee stated that investments would have to be realised to meet the purchase price, but obviously the money was available. Negotiations were completed within the year and the new offices were opened by Princess Mary, Viscountess Lascelles, on April 20th, 1925, after a short prayer of dedication by the Archdeacon of London. Following this, the full Council was able to meet, for the first time in its own premises. In October 1927, however, it was announced that "the present house would not be sufficient for the Council's needs for more than five years, if so long" and the Minister of Health was informed.

FINANCE

The registration of existing and intermediate nurses provided the Council with sufficient capital to acquire worthwhile investments. These brought in a small income. In 1924, Council decided that nurses registering by virtue of examination should not be required to pay an initial registration fee, but simply the annual retention fee. The accounts were audited annually: in 1924 the balance was £16,412. At no time could the Council feel complacent about its finance since costs and expenditure continued to rise, while income was difficult to estimate since it depended largely on the numbers paying the annual retention fee and taking examinations.

THE SELECT COMMITTEE 1925

Due to pressure from various bodies and individuals, the Minister set up a Select Committee of the House of Commons in 1925 to "consider the Rules of the General Nursing Council with regard to the prescribed training for nurses and the reservation of seats on the Council for matrons." The members of the committee were Major Sir Richard Barnett, Sir George Berry, Mr. Rhys Davies, Mr. Fisher, Colonel Fremantle, Sir Charles Forestier Walker, Mr. Hurst, Major-General Sir Richard Luce, Colonel Sinclair, Miss Wilkinson, and Mr. Robert Wilson. The committee held seven meetings and called fifteen witnesses representing the Ministry of Health, the General Nursing

Council, The College of Nursing, The Royal British Nurses' Association, the Professional Union of Trained Nurses, the Registered Nurses' Parliamentary Council, and matrons, sister tutors and other nurses.

Each witness was questioned as to:

(i) Whether the Rules proposed by the General Nursing Council in regard to the prescribed training for nurses in fact comply with the provisions of the Act.

(ii) What is the best method of securing that a proper and adequate training shall be obtained by all nurses applying for Registration?

(iii) What is the best scheme of election that can be prescribed under the provisions of the Schedule to the Act.

As regards points (i) and (ii) witnesses either wished to make the training syllabus compulsory, or were happy with the syllabus of examination. Those who spoke in favour of a compulsory training syllabus were Mrs. Fenwick; Miss Philpott, A.R.R.C., Matron of High Wycombe and District War Memorial Hospital, an affiliated training school; Miss du Sautoy, a member of the General Nursing Council; Miss Macdonald, Secretary of the Royal British Nurses' Association; Councillor Beatrice Kent, President of the Registered Nurses' Parliamentary Council; Miss Pearce, an L.C.C. Superintendent of School Nurses; and Miss MacCallum, Hon. Secretary of the Professional Union of Trained Nurses. Two witnesses liked the training syllabus but wanted it to be advisory: Miss E. Innes, R.R.C., Matron of the General Infirmary at Leeds who represented the College of Nursing; and Miss L. Duff Grant, Sister Tutor at the General Infirmary at Leeds. Those who preferred the examination syllabus were: Sir Wilmot Herringham; Miss M. C. Herbert, Sister Tutor, St. George-in-the-East Hospital, London (the champion of the bona fide nurses); and Miss Kate Heywood, Matron of Walthamstow, Wanstead and Leyton Children's and General Hospital, an associated training school.

Mr. Patterson, a surgeon, did not like either syllabus and wanted a new one!

As regards the election, only three people spoke in favour of keeping "reserved seats" for matrons on the Council: they were Sir Wilmot Herringham, Miss Heywood and Miss Philpott. Everyone else wanted "free" elections. Many of the witnesses were very vocal and expressed opinions outside the matters on which they were asked. However, the Committee completed its work in under six weeks and published its conclusions, which were:

(1) The word training (in the Act) does not necessarily involve a scheme of training more detailed than that which is prescribed in the Rules and the syllabus of examination together with the nurses' chart.

(2) It did not recommend that the training syllabus should be made compulsory, but it was impressed with the value of such a scheme as a guide to training—it should not be withdrawn. The Committee members were against a more elementary syllabus, and might have been quoting Miss Nightingale when they said "the minimum usually tends to become a maximum, and the high standard set by the present syllabus, once lowered, would be very difficult to work up to again."

(3) It felt that insufficient protection was afforded to probationer nurses, in that too much of their time was being absorbed with the ordinary work of the hospital. The General Nursing Council were asked to look into this and to take steps to ensure that all probationers be guaranteed a minimum number of student hours.

(4) It was impressed with the need for inspection of training schools and recommended that the General Nursing Council carry out their expressed intention in this matter without delay.

(5) Over the election, it was impressed with the importance of the Council's educational duties and thought these must have first place in considering the Constitution (even though they realised the disciplinary function). It recommended that at the next election there should be a free vote for the eleven "general" seats.

The Select Committee highlighted many problems of nurse training which still exist and this is well illustrated by the following exchange between the Chairman of the Committee, Mr. Fisher, and Mr. Brock, who represented the Ministry of Health.

"*Mr. Fisher.* That is where the difficulty arises, is it not, that the probationer is both a student and a worker in the hospital, and the claims to some extent conflict?

Mr. Brock. Yes, and there is always the temptation to a hospital to try and get more work than it is fair to get out of a student.

Mr. Fisher. The problem really is a problem of adjusting the frontiers between these two claims?

Mr. Brock. It is a very difficult problem indeed"[15].

PERSONALITIES

Few people realise how much work and time may be involved in being a member of the General Nursing Council. In the early days this must have been particularly so since the foundations for the future were being laid. In 1923 it appears that both Committees and Council were very overworked, and one member commented "towards the end of a Committee Meeting we sit with fixed eyes, glaring at one another and saying no, when we mean yes"[16]. One can sympathise, while hoping this did not happen too often! As previously mentioned, Miss Ellen Musson had resigned from her matron's post, on learning of her election and Miss Cox-Davies had done so too, during the caretaker Council. These two were to play a leading part in the Council's affairs for the next two decades, and it is obvious that Miss Musson was seen as a suitable Chairman by Sir Wilmot Herringham since, in his statement at the January Council meeting in 1926, he said Miss Musson was now ready to stand and had been training herself for that particular position. In consequence he was not willing to stand for nomination. There was therefore only one candidate before the Council and there would be no need for a ballot. Miss Musson agreed to take the Chair and she and several other Council members thanked Sir Wilmot for all he had done. Almost six years after the first Council Meeting, a nurse was elected Chairman of the statutory body and this has continued ever since. Mrs. Fenwick was delighted, since she had always felt—and said—that nurses should take the lead in their own affairs. She devoted two and a half columns of the Editorial of the current *British Journal of Nursing* to the event, and called the announcement one of momentous significance. The *Nursing Times* called it a tribute to the successful work of State Registration.

Sir Wilmot Herringham became vice-Chairman until the next election.

APPROVAL OF TRAINING SCHOOLS

During 1926 and 1927 the Council came into conflict with the Ministry over the approval of two hospitals as training schools. In both cases the dispute arose because the Council felt the hospitals to be too small and to have inadequate clinical material.

In the case of Darlington Isolation Hospital, the hospital authorities appealed to the Minister under Section 7 of the Nurses Registration Act 1919 and the Minister allowed the appeal. He directed the Council to approve the hospital as a complete training school for fever nurses, subject to the condition that, except with the consent of the Council, there should not be more than ten probationers training at the institution at any one time. The Minister said that Darlington was representative of the smaller hospitals, and the real question was, could the training provided in hospitals of this type, reasonably be regarded as adequate. He thought that the clinical material available should be considered in relation to the number of probationers. He argued that the Fever Hospitals Association were unlikely to accept too sudden a change in its training methods. The Council accepted the Minister's decision and altered its normal rule of a minimum of 40 occupied beds, for fever hospitals, to 38 beds so as to approve Darlington. Nine months later, another fever hospital appealed to the Minister. Hastings Infectious Diseases Hospital had been approved as a training school by the Fever Nurses' Association in 1923, with the result that it was found much easier to obtain probationers of a better standard. In 1926, as the Fever Nurses' Association had come to an end, the hospital authorities applied to the General Nursing Council for recognition as a complete training for the fever Register. This had been refused. The hospital consisted of 12 wards in four separate blocks totalling 70 beds, and an operating theatre, and according to the authorities, treatment was on modern lines. The nursing staff consisted of a matron, two sisters, two staff nurses and six probationers. The hospital authorities' case was that the clinical experience was adequate and that lack of approval meant they would have greater difficulties in getting probationers; they contended that it was quite possible to give nurses as good a training with a small number of cases in a small hospital, as with a larger number in a larger institution.

The Council's case was that there had to be a minimum number of occupied beds: fever hospitals had only been recognised with a minimum of 40 occupied beds except for Darlington which was just under 40. In the Hastings case the number was only 15 and the Council could not come down to that: 15 occupied beds was not sufficient to constitute a complete training school although it could constitute an affiliated training school. In response to a question one of the Hastings doctors admitted that 82 per cent of the cases in the previous year were of only two types—scarlet fever and diphtheria—(and only seven patients in the year had diphtheria). These facts all emerged at an enquiry held at the Ministry of Health. The result was as follows:

"The Minister, after consideration of the matter, and in the exercise of powers conferred on him by the said Section (7, Nurses Registration Act) affirms the decision of the Council, but directs that the Council shall give the hospital approval as a complete training school for fever nurses, in the case of all probationers who are now serving in it or who may enter it before July 1st, 1934 (seven years later) subject to the following conditions:

(1) A probationer shall not be qualified to sit for the Final Examination until she has completed a three years' course of training (normally two years).

(2) The approval shall have effect so long only as the number of the staff other than probationers does not fall below the number so employed on March 15th, 1927."

When this was announced, the Chairman—Miss Musson—said that the Council had no power to question the decision but it was referred to the Education and Examinations Committee.

In November a special meeting of Council was held to discuss the Hastings case. The Education and Examination Committee asked Council to note that it believed it to be a dangerous precedent. They pointed out the reasons for the existence of the General Nursing Council, its Constitution and powers, its position with regard to the fever hospitals and the existing affiliation schemes for small hospitals. They were particularly concerned at the decision to˙increase the length of training, which was apparently an attempt to make up for the deficiency of clinical material. Every member of Council spoke in support of a resolution which was drawn up and sent to the Minister which said, "the General Nursing Council desires to offer a strong protest against the decision of the Minister of Health . . . which in the Council's opinion not only permits a totally insufficient training in this particular hospital, but will by its effect prevent an adequate standard from being maintained. The Council instructs its representatives to solicit a further interview to enable it to state the facts to the Minister himself."

In this attitude the Council was supported by the Fever Nurses' Association, the College of Nursing, the Association of Hospital Matrons, the British College of Nurses, and the Northern Ireland Joint Nursing and Midwives Council. However, the same reply was sent to all bodies who wrote complaining about the decision: "in reply, I am to point out, that the General Nursing Council and the Town Council placed their views fully before the Minister . . . at the hearing of the appeal . . . and his decision was given after exhaustive consideration of the issue from every point of view . . . the Minister is exercising an appellate jurisdiction and he cannot undertake to discuss . . . a decision given by him in his judicial capacity under Section 7 of the Nurses Registration Act 1919". No further hearing was granted to the Council's representatives.

THE ELECTION 1927

Before the Select Committee met in 1925 the Council had submitted a scheme for the next election, with reserved seats for matrons and the Minister had signed this. However, once the Committee report was published, an amended scheme was drawn up, and signed. This provided for eleven seats open to all on the general Register, and five seats distributed in the same way as before for the supplementary Registers.

Once again, the College held meetings and published lists of approved candidates. The *Nursing Times* wrote "It is a matter of history that independent candidates stand less chance of election than those having the support of organisations behind them"[17]. Mrs. Fenwick was asked to stand again, but refused. She wrote, in the *British Journal of Nursing*, "the majority of nurses in this kingdom are too ignorant of nursing politics and too subject to economic control and to financial patronage, to give a free vote for candidates"[18].

The College recommended twelve candidates—eleven for the general seats and one for the male nurses seat, although at this this time, male nurses could not be College members. All twelve were elected. As before, only those independent candidates standing for the supplementary Registers were returned. The elected nurses were:

General nurses:	votes	
Alicia Lloyd Still	13,406	
Margaret Elwin Sparshott	13,366	
Rachael Annie Cox-Davies	12,363	
Ellen Mary Musson	11,260	
Harriet Amelia Alsop	10,951	
Geraldine Bremner	10,704	
Letitia Sarah Clark	10,130	Matron, Whipps Cross Hospital
Marion Agnes Gullan	10,009	Sister Tutor, St. Thomas's Hospital
Margaret Hogg	9,302	Matron, Guy's Hospital
Gertrude Cowlin	8,410	(Now Editor, *Nursing Times*)
Emily Meadows	6,968	Sister, University College Hospital

Female mental nurses, Jean Brown, 1,475
Male mental nurses, Edwin Robert Blackman, 1,561
Sick Children's nurses, Alice Mary Bushby, 336
Male nurses, Frederick William Stratton (unopposed)
Fever nurses, Susan Villiers (unopposed).

Of the general nurses four members were new and of the nurses representing the supplementary Registers the two mental nurses were new.

On December 16th, 1927 the first elected Council met for the last time and the Chairman, Miss Musson, gave a short review of the work of the last five years: she ended by saying "perhaps one of the notable changes which has taken place during one term of office has been that every chair, but one, has latterly been occupied by a Registered Nurse".

COMPARISONS

Those readers, who at this point, feel concern at some of the difficulties and problems that have been recorded, may be interested and perhaps reassured to compare some details of the Council's history with those of another organisation. The early days of the G.N.C. may be compared with the early days of the General Medical Council which finally came into being after eighteen years of parliamentary debate. Between 1840 and 1858, seventeen medical Bills were introduced and foundered, before the first Medical Act received the Royal Assent on August 2nd, 1858.

The first meeting of the General Medical Council was held on November 23rd, 1858 and the problems they faced were similar to those experienced by the General Nursing Council. Before the Act was passed, there were nineteen separate Licensing Bodies for doctors and some of the titles conferred had purely local value. The Census returns of 1841 suggested that of 15,000 doctors who were practising, 5,000 were completely unqualified. The G.M.C. recorded in 1869 that "in the main body of the profession, those to whom the main bulk of the population must always look for medical assistance, the education was so defective that the profession was in danger of being overrun with illiterate and incompetent men".

The successful Act had involved compromises and laid down principles rather than detail; it authorised the Council to compile and publish an annual Register and all those practising in 1815 (having therefore 43 years practice) were admitted to the Register even if they had no qualification. The unregistered were not forbidden to practice, but could not claim that they were registered.

Parliament had underestimated the difficulties of forming a Register for doctors. The Act had foreseen the publication of the Register at the beginning of 1859, but like the nurses, thousands of doctors left it to the last minute to apply and because of this, an Amending Act had to be passed postponing the limitations on unregistered doctors.

In July 1859 the first Register was published and contained nearly 15,000 names. Subsequent numbers are as follows:

1880   23,000 names
1924   50,000 names
1958   90,000 names

The first G.M.C. had 24 members representing the 19 Licensing Bodies—many of whom disagreed strongly with each other. One eminent physician said, "much fighting is anticipated, but I look for better things", and another member of Council wrote that "divergencies had been not seldom expressed in language requiring the moderating influence of the chairman"[19].

References

1. *Nursing Times*—6.1.23.
2. *British Journal of Nursing*—3.2.23.
3. *Nursing Times*—21.4.23.
4. Ibid.—12.5.23.
5. Ibid.—23.6.23.
6. *British Journal of Nursing*—30.6.23.
7. *Nursing Times*—21.7.23.
8. A History of the Nursing Profession, p. 111. Abel Smith.
9. *Nursing Times*—10.11.23.
10. Ibid.—14.6.24.
11. Ibid.—9.8.24.
12. Ibid.—15.1.27.
13. Ibid.—23.5.25.
14. Ibid.—14.7.28.
15. Select Committee on the G.N.C.—1925.
16. *Nursing Times*—14.4.23.
17. Ibid.—1.10.27.
18. *British Journal of Nursing*—November 1927.
19. Centenary of the General Medical Council 1858–1958, Pyke-Lees.

Chapter 6

1928–1938

"The common problem, yours, mine, everyones
Is not to fancy what were fair in life
Provided it could be;—but finding first
What may be, then find how to make it fair
Up to our means—a very different thing!"   BROWNING

At the beginning of 1928 the appointed members of the new Council were announced. They were:

Board of Education: Miss Eleanor Wilson
John Fawcett, M.D., F.R.C.P., F.R.C.S.

Privy Council: Lady Galway, C.B.E.
Miss E. S. Haldane, C.H., LL.D., J.P.

Ministry of Health: Lady Barrett
Dr. J. J. Buchan, D.P.H.
Rev. G. B. Cronshaw
Dr. F. H. Thomson, D.P.H.
Dr. R. Worth, C.B.E.

According to the nursing press, all the newly appointed members were directly, or indirectly connected with the nursing profession; this was an interesting comment, since the Act specifically stated that the two Privy Council nominees should not have anything to do with nursing or medicine!

At the first meeting of the new Council on January 20th, 1928 Miss Musson, who had been re-elected Chairman, was congratulated on being awarded the C.B.E. in the New Years Honours List. The new vice-Chairman was Miss Cox-Davies. The returning officer stated that at the recent election 50,502 voting papers had been sent out, 21,188 were returned in time and 483 were invalid. During the next decade, this and the next Council (1932), continued and developed the now familiar routine work of approval of training schools, examinations, registration and discipline. In addition to this, several major events called for a rethinking or change in policy.

93

THE MENTAL NURSES

In 1926 the Council had ceased to recognise the R.M.P.A. certificate for Registration as a Mental Nurse. Early in 1928 the Scottish General Nursing Council wrote to the R.M.P.A. and suggested that the qualifying examinations for both bodies should be conducted jointly. A leading Scottish psychiatrist, Professor Robertson, did not think that the existing Preliminary Examination was suitable for nurses taking mental training; he also said that the Act gave the Councils power to delegate responsibility for examinations to another body—e.g. the R.M.P.A. The English Mental Nurses Committee felt that it would be best for a joint conference of the three Councils to be held to discuss the matter, since reciprocity could only be possible if all were agreed on major decisions regarding training.

Mental nurses themselves were divided and letters on the subject were published in the press throughout 1928 and 1929. Those who were in favour of the Council's examinations continually stressed the fact that the R.M.P.A. was a purely medical body and as such should not have a controlling voice in nurse training; one wrote "the chief reason why mental nurses are not entering for the State Examination is simply that medical superintendents are so obviously imbued and contented with the old regime"[1].

Others however, felt that the R.M.P.A. was just as good as the General Nursing Council and wanted a mental nurses' sub-committee of experts including doctors, matrons and nurses.

On June 23rd, 1928 the conference between the three Councils was held. It is perhaps interesting to note that at this time neither the Chairman of the Scottish nor the Northern Ireland Council was a nurse. The conference reached four conclusions:

(1) The higher fees charged by the three State Nursing Councils appeared to be one reason why mental nurses were taking the R.M.P.A. rather than the Councils' examinations.

(2) It was decided unanimously to continue with the same Preliminary Examination for the general and supplementary parts of the Register.

(3) It was debatable whether it was legally permissible under

the Act, for the Councils to accept the examinations of any outside body.

(4) It was decided to continue with the existing method of appointing examiners for mental nurses.

The conference were unanimous in their belief that the advantages of being State Registered had not been explained fully to nurses in many mental hospitals, and passed a resolution saying that it was impossible for them to accept the certificate of another examining body, outside themselves, for the purposes of registration.

In September, the National Asylum Workers' Union held a conference and passed a resolution, "that this conference instructs its members on the General Nursing Council to use all their efforts to obtain State Registration for all holders of the R.M.P.A. certificate". Miss Wiese had hoped the conference would reject the resolution but arrived too late to oppose it; it was not, however, a unanimous decision[2]. At the same time the R.M.P.A. issued a report based on a questionnaire sent to all training schools for mental nurses: of 104, recognised by the General Nursing Council, 60 prepared candidates for the State Examinations and 51 had actually entered candidates.

The Mental Hospital Matrons' Association passed a resolution warmly supporting the two examinations conducted by the General Nursing Council and urging mental nurses to enter for these examinations which were run by a body representing the nurses themselves.

A letter in the press at this time said "we have reached a critical stage in the development of mental nursing. The question is not merely one of State Registration: the issues are wider and more significant. . . . Are the nurses in a mental hospital under the control of the matron, or do they work directly under the Medical Superintendent?"[3]. On the same theme, Miss Macaulay wrote to say that a great advantage of the Councils' examination was that the oral and practical parts were conducted entirely by nurses. She objected to the medical profession tampering with the Nurses Registration Act and pointed out that the General Nursing Council's Certificate had legal status while the R.M.P.A.'s had not. "Why cannot the R.M.P.A. withdraw gracefully, as the old order must inevitably give place to the new".[4]

As a result of the controversy the Council decided to take Counsels opinion on the relevant point about examinations in the Act.

In the Spring of 1929 members of the General Nursing Council met a delegation from the R.M.P.A. headed by Professor Robertson. The R.M.P.A. felt that so far the Council's examination for the mental register was a failure, since so few were taking it. They were prepared to accept the Council's syllabus of training and inspection of their (the R.M.P.A.'s) examinations, if the Council were prepared to accept the R.M.P.A. certificate for registration. Miss Musson, for the Council, said that to make the nursing profession, or any branch of it, dependent for its status on another profession, would be to give up the rights that had been won for them by an Act of Parliament. Although both sides were obviously sincere, they could not reach agreement.

Questions were asked in the House of Commons, and the Minister, Mr. Greenwood, said that he felt that the matter could be adjusted by the two bodies concerned.

Early in 1930 a private member, Mr. J. R. Remer, tried to introduce a Nurses Registration Act Amendment Bill to enable nurses possessing the R.M.P.A. certificate to register as mental nurses. However, this did not succeed, and in reply to a question to the Minister as to whether he intended to amend the 1919 Act, the reply was "No Sir".

At about the same time, representatives of the Mental Nurses Committee of the General Nursing Council met representatives of the Mental Hospitals Association; both groups again stated the same viewpoints but Miss Musson, for the Council, was adamant that only one body could set up examinations to achieve a common standard for the Register, and that body was the Council.

At the Autumn meeting of the National Asylum Workers' Union, a resolution was carried urging that a separate register for mental nurses should be established under the control of the Mental Hospitals Association, the R.M.P.A. and the Union[5]. However, nothing came of this and although the problem was not solved, things continued as they were for two years.

In 1932, the Mental Nurses Committee of the General Nursing Council wrote to the R.M.P.A. thanking them for their help and advice through the Advisory Committee on examinations, and suggesting that as the latter had not met for six years, it should now be dissolved.

It is obvious that the concern felt by nurses over the control of mental hospitals was to some extent justified, since in June 1933 the Mental Nurses Committee reported that a letter had been received from the Mental Hospitals Matrons' Association, to the effect that a matron with no nursing qualification had been appointed at a mental nurse training school. Approval was subsequently withdrawn from this hospital until the position was rectified.

During the 1930s, the number entering for the Council's Final Examination for the Mental and Mental Defective parts of the Register remained small, some 40–60 sitting on each occasion. The R.M.P.A. continued to run its own examinations and discussions and correspondence went on in a desultory fashion.

INSPECTION OF TRAINING SCHOOLS

The question of the need for the Council to inspect nurse-training schools had been raised during the hearing of the 1925 Select Committee and the Committee had recommended "that the Council should carry out its expressed intention in this matter". It was decided to implement this as soon as possible and the matter was referred to the Education and Examinations Committee. Over the next 18 months, members of Council began making visits to training schools, particularly those seeking approval. Miss Musson and Miss Lloyd Still paid visits to the Ministry of Health to discuss a scheme and an informal conference was held with representatives of the British Hospitals Association, the Board of Control and the Association of Poor Law Unions all of whom seemed quite happy with the proposed arrangements.

In June 1928 a draft scheme of inspection was forwarded to the Ministry of Health. A reply was received from the Ministry a month later. The Minister (Mr. Neville Chamberlain) could not agree to the scheme since he was not happy about the position of Poor Law Infirmaries, as these were already inspected by his staff and he was not convinced that this should be done twice.

The correspondence continued, and those members of Council who could give time, visited training schools. Legal opinion was taken and the Council's solicitor, Mr. Sidney Pitt, stated that the Council could not read any legal right of inspection into the Registration Act. In February 1929 a further letter was sent to the Minister; it stated that the Nurses Registration Act had made approval of training schools one of the Council's duties, and this could not be done except with first hand knowledge—in fact for some time, no voluntary general, children's or fever hospital had been approved until it had been visited by a member of Council. In the Registration Act, no difference had been made between voluntary and public or municipal hospitals.

Little progress was made, despite a deputation to the Ministry, partly due to the changes in hospital administration envisaged under the Local Government Act of 1929. However, as nothing more had been heard by 1931, Council wrote asking for another meeting at the Ministry. At this visit Miss Musson pointed out that the scheme could not start until the Minister sanctioned payment for expenses. The Ministry officials suggested that Council should now write to them on two separate issues, one asking for money and the other regarding the Council's right to inspect all hospitals. This correspondence continued and two of the appointed members tried to obtain private interviews with the Minister. By July 1932 Miss Musson suggested that Council should write to the Minister saying that as they had been unable to obtain an interview, they had decided to carry out the proposed scheme. As a result the Minister saw a deputation in his room at the House of Commons but no further progress was made over the Poor Law Hospitals.

Three years later, in 1935, at another meeting with Ministry officials, Miss Musson pointed out that Council had been waiting for a decision since 1927. She said that at present, she and three other Council members, no longer in active work, were doing what visits they could but this could not continue indefinitely.

Having still made no progress by the spring of 1936, Council decided to finance a limited scheme of visits out of its own investments. It was agreed that a small number of registered nurses, who had held posts as matrons of hospitals approved by the Council, be invited to assist as and when required. Two well-known nurses, Miss Hogg (ex-Matron of Guy's and ex-member of Council) and Miss Montgomery (ex-Matron of the Middlesex Hospital) were approached and agreed to do this. A scheme was drawn up by which, it was hoped, each training school would be visited once in five years, and the visitors were asked to make recommendations to the Council, who would forward a report to the authorities concerned. Before the new arrangements, four or five hospitals had been visited each month, now the number was more than doubled. Although no official sanction had been given, some Poor Law Hospitals were included—often on the authorities' invitation—and visits were sometimes discussed with the Ministry's Inspectors.

In 1938 Miss Montgomery withdrew through illness and two further ex-matrons joined Miss Hogg: they were Miss Lloyd, ex-Matron of Lancaster Royal Infirmary and Miss Cockeram, ex-Matron of Birmingham Children's Hospital and ex-member of Council.

Finally, owing to the onset of war in 1939 it was officially decided that there should be "co-operation between the Ministry of Health and the General Nursing Council in the matters of visits of inspection to recognised Public Assistance Hospitals so that the report on the visit of either body should also serve the purposes of the other".

As Miss Musson had said, in 1932, regarding the question of inspections "the Council feel that only time and patience can remove this and some other difficulties". Perhaps she should have added—"or a war".

THE LANCET COMMISSION REPORT

In 1930 a commission was set up by the proprietors of the *Lancet* to "inquire into the reasons for the shortage of candidates, trained and untrained, for nursing the sick in general and special hospitals throughout the country, and to offer suggestions for making the service more attractive to women suitable for this necessary work". The final report was published in January 1932. No member of the General Nursing Council was on this commission and the majority of its findings had nothing to do with the Council's statutory duties. However, some recommendations were concerned with training:

(a) Means of overcoming the "gap"; that is the period between leaving school and being able to start nurse-training (paras 65–99).

(b) Alternative methods of meeting the cost of training by scholarships, etc. (paras 102–122).

(c) The Preliminary Examination should be divided into two halves: Part 1, dealing with anatomy, physiology and hygiene; Part 2 with the theory and practice of nursing; the General Nursing Council should recognise centres where Part 1 could be taken, not more than two years before entering training—e.g., secondary schools. Alternatively, anyone with a degree or advanced examination in these subjects should be exempt from Part 1.

The questions in the Final Examination should be confined to nursing treatment and should not involve systematic medicine, surgery, gynaecology or psychiatry. Hospitals should release a nurse from duty at least on the day before, as well as the day of her Final written and oral examinations. Sister-tutors should be provided in a ratio of 1-60 students and not be required to undertake duties other than those connected with education (paras 215–241)

(d) Recognition of previous training; the General Nursing Council should empower all hospitals approved as complete training schools to make allowance for time spent in other approved schools (paras 243–252).

(e) Staffing of non-approved hospitals. Hospitals not approved by the General Nursing Council should not seek to enlist probationers for training (paras 281–285).

(f) Mental hospitals. There is an urgent need for general hospitals to accept Registered Mental Nurses for a two year training as recommended by the General Nursing Council (paras 308–336).

The commission also discussed other questions of policy outside its terms of reference, among which were the establishment of schools of nursing connected with universities for higher grades, even if not for basic training, and the need for two grades of trained nurse.

From the General Nursing Council's point of view, the most controversial of these recommendations was the proposal to "split the Prelim" and this concept played a large part in both the 1932 and 1937 elections for the Council for England and Wales.

"SPLITTING THE PRELIM"

In June 1932, the Scottish General Nursing Council passed a resolution to divide the Preliminary Examination into two parts, as suggested by the *Lancet* Commission. In reply to a letter from the Council for England and Wales, deprecating this new departure without consultation, the Scottish Registrar wrote saying that no steps had yet been taken to put the resolution into effect.

At about the same time the College of Nursing wrote to the Council saying they were in favour of the proposed division and in its answer the Council said that they had no authority to recognise secondary schools; they had no objection to the inclusion, in the school curriculum, of some of the subjects necessary for the Preliminary Examination, but felt that in principle, the continuation of a broad, general education was preferable.

Letters appeared in the nursing press both for and against the division of the examination.

At the end of the year the Council had discussions on the subject with their opposite numbers in Scotland and with officials of the Ministry, and all parties decided to defer further consultation for six months.

A comment in the *British Journal of Nursing* is interesting: "the value of lectures on anatomy, physiology and hygiene taken in conjunction with nursing practice and experience and directly related thereto is infinitely greater than if it is regarded merely from an academic point of view"[6]. This of course is the basis of the 1962 syllabus.

Early in 1933 the new Education and Examinations Committee postponed the whole question until September. At the November Council meeting the matter was fully debated: three letters and a memorandum were noted. A letter from the Royal British Nurses' Association said there were grave dangers in the division; one from the Headmistresses' Association said their executive committee would welcome the new proposal; and one from the National Council of Women, agreed with Headmistresses. The memorandum (stimulated by Miss Innes) was from prominent medical men in Leeds and urged that no division should take place. The Education and Examinations Committee put forward a resolution saying that division would not be in the best interest of the candidates or the profession— after discussion, this was agreed, 9–5. Mr. Eason (a nominated member) moved an amendment that the examination should be divided: voting for this was 11 for—13 against. The resolution was therefore carried as it stood.

Correspondence on the subject continued in the national and professional press and between the General Nursing Councils for Scotland and for England and Wales.

In May 1934, Middlesex County Council wrote to the General Nursing Council with a suggested two-year pre-nursing course. The Council answered saying that the course would be very helpful to a girl who was going to take up nursing; however, they suggested that one year's further general education and one year of specialised subjects would be better, and they could not agree to any statutory examination being taken at the end of the course.

Since a majority of the Council were not in favour of this change, nothing further happened till 1937, except that the Scottish Council decided to draft an amendment to the Rules allowing the examination to be divided. At the end of 1937 the elections (in England and Wales) resulted in a Council, with ten new elected nurses, and at the Council meeting in March 1938 a resolution was passed "that the Council approve of the division of the Preliminary State Examination into two parts: Part 1 of the examination, which may be taken before entry to a training school, shall include the subjects of anatomy, physiology and hygiene. A candidate taking Part 1 of the Examination before entrance to a training school will be required to produce evidence that she has undergone a course of instruction approved by the General Nursing Council which shall include the above subjects. The minimum age of entry to Part 1 of the examination shall be 18 years. The Education and Examination Committee are requested to submit draft regulations for giving effect to this resolution."

The resolution which was moved by Miss Dey, and amended by Miss MacManus was discussed fully. Most of the members were in favour but one point of argument was whether the courses should be full or part time. Miss Musson however said "as you all know I am not in favour". Her objection was the divorce of two practical subjects from the curriculum; she "very much approved" of pre-nursing courses, but felt it was a pity that one of a nurse's professional examinations, which was part of her training, should take place before she entered a training school.

By the end of the year, the draft Rule for "splitting the Prelim" was approved for submission to the Minister of Health. Candidates had to:

pass the entrance test (page 198) either before entry, or
within three months of entry, or
have passed the Matriculation examination, or　　　　a
have School Certificate of Boards listed, or
have passed some examination approved by the Council.

OR

May enter for Part, 1 after a course approved by the
Council, or　　　　b
on completion of not less than six months in a
training school.

The entrance fee was to be £1 10s. for each part and £2 2s. if both parts were taken together. The minimum age for entry to Part 1 was $17\frac{1}{2}$ years.

The Rules were signed in 1939, and one of the first schools to be approved for a course leading to Part 1 was Cheltenham Ladies College. The first "divided" Part 1 was held in December 1939 and there were 35 candidates.

THE 1932 ELECTION

Two main issues governed the 1932 election: the College of Nursing were especially keen that everyone should state their views on the Preliminary Examination, and the *British Journal of Nursing* wanted to know whether this would be the last time the College would dominate an election!

The *Nursing Times* editorial of October 1st said, "there is a vital need to elect those who agree with "Splitting the Prelim". We need to choose leaders who can make easy contact with leaders in other kindred professions—women with uncanny foresight and with the strength and courage to shape our affairs according to what they see"[7].

Nineteen candidates stood for the eleven "general "seats. At a meeting to hear their views, the joint committee of the College of Nursing, the Association of Hospital Matrons and the County and County Borough Hospital Matrons' Association chose twelve candidates and asked the voters to elect eleven of these. Of the twelve chosen, one was a sister-tutor, one a public health tutor, five were matrons (three of London teaching hospitals) and five were ex-matrons (one of a London teaching hospital). An ex-matron wrote to the *Nursing Times* and said "no less than fifteen of the candidates standing for elections are either existing, or ex-matrons". She appreciated the importance of their work but felt that other interests had an equal right to representation on the Council. "It would be most unfortunate if the General Nursing Council should eventually become a kind of "retiring-shelf" in perpetuity for those no longer in active nursing, since they must in the nature of things, as time goes on, lose touch with current opinion on important points"[8].

For the supplementary registers, four male candidates stood, three male and three female mental nurses, two sick children's nurses, and the fever nurses' candidate was unopposed.

The successful candidates were:

General nurses:	*votes*	
Alicia Lloyd Still	12,681	re-elected
Rachael A. Cox-Davies	11,610	re-elected
Margaret E. Sparshott	11,084	re-elected
Emily E. P. MacManus	10,256	Matron, Guy's
Ellen M. Musson	10,160	re-elected
Euphemia S. Innes	10,054	Matron, General Infirmary, Leeds
Helen Dey	9,575	Matron, St. Bartholomew's
Mary Jones	8,566	Matron, Liverpool Royal Infirmary
Marion Agnes Gullan	8,203	re-elected
Winifred Bowling	7,418	Matron, Royal Infirmary, Sheffield
Ruth Darbyshire	7,415	Matron, University College Hospital

Female mental:
    Kathleen M. Willis   1,013   St. Lawrence Hospital,
                                     Caterham

Male mental:
    John Henry Buckley   1,093   Charge Nurse, Three
                                     Counties Hospital, Beds

Sick Children's:
    Edith Cockeram   436   Matron Children's
                                     Hospital, Birmingham

Male nurses:
    John Southwell   50

Fever nurses:
    Susan Villiers   —   Unopposed

The press commented that the new Council was not unanimous in its convictions, but that it would be vigorous. More seriously, the total omission of any representative from the general Municipal Hospitals and the Public Health field was noted.

The returning officer stated that 62,970 voting papers had been sent out, 21,775 returned in time (approximately 35 per cent) and 263 were invalid.

The nominated members were:

Privy Council: Countess of Limerick
                           Viscountess Erleigh (Daughter of Mr. Alfred Mond, Minister of Health in the early 1920s)

Board of Education: Miss Gwatkin (Headmistress, Streatham Hill High School)
                           Mrs. J. S. Courtauld

Ministry of Health: Mr. Harper (House Governor, Wolverhampton Royal Hospital)
                           Mr. Eason (Medical Superintendent, Guy's Hospital)
                           Dr. M. A. Collins (Medical

Superintendent, Kent County Mental
Hospital)
Dr. Margaret Kettle (Assistant
Editor of the *Lancet*)
Dr. Porter (Medical Officer of
Health)

THE REGISTRAR

In September 1933, Miss Riddell's forthcoming retirement
was announced: it will be remembered that she was the General
Nursing Council's first Registrar and had taken up her appointment in the early days of the Caretaker Council. On January
26th, 1934, a presentation was made to Miss Riddell at 20
Portland Place: the gift consisted of two armchairs and a
settee. Miss Musson said "it is many years since a little Scottish
probationer was sent up to my ward. A very good little probationer she was—conscientious, hardworking, a little apt to be
worried sometimes, always generous and kind hearted as she is
today." She went on to say, the time had come, as it comes to
us all, when Miss Riddell wanted more leisure, some of it for
her garden. Jewellery had seemed to the givers a less useful idea
than something comfortable, and so she (Miss Musson) would
just ask Miss Riddell to take the Chair, and suiting the action
to the word, gently propelled her forward on to the settee. Miss
Riddell thanked everyone for this provision for her old age,
and could not wish her successor anything better than the unfailing help and loyalty she herself had enjoyed all these years.'

An official appreciation was recorded in the Council's
minutes.

The new Registrar, who took up her appointment at the
beginning of 1934 was Miss Gwladys Evelyn Davies, S.R.N.
Miss Davies trained at the Royal Southern Hospital, Liverpool
from 1907–10, and subsequently held the appointment of Night
Sister at the Royal Hospital, Richmond. During the 1914–18
war she served in England, France and Serbia. Before joining
the Council's staff she was sister-in-charge of the out-patient
department at the South London Hospital for Women. In 1920
she became the General Nursing Council's Registration Officer
and after a short break became Assistant Registrar in June
1924.

There had been 24 applicants for the post and this time the Council had not fixed any definite age limit in connection with the appointment.

THE RETENTION FEE AND FINANCE

The difficulty in collecting the annual retention fee continued to be one of the Council's problems: for example, in 1928, 51,661 forms were issued and 47,659 fees were received. During the late '20s and early '30s there was some feeling that the retention fee should be abolished and letters to this effect appeared in the press.

In March 1931 the Council issued a statement explaining its position; it pointed out the wording of the Act, "there shall be paid to the Council in respect of every application . . . to be registered . . . and in respect of the retention in any year of any person on the Register, such fees as the Council may, with the approval of the Minister of Health, from time to time determine". The main reason for an annual fee was to keep a "live" Register and many people rang the Council to check on Registered nurses. Changes of address and of names—due to marriage—were approximately 15,000 a year out of 60,000 on the Register and these were usually notified when the retention fee was paid. It was pointed out that payment was easy: a reminder was sent on August 31st each year; if the fee had not been received by October 31st a second reminder was issued, and if it had still not been received by November 30th the name was removed from the Register. The Register had to be published each year under the Act. The Council reminded nurses that under the Act of 1858, doctors paid no annual fee but their initial registration fee was £5; dentists however, whose Act was in 1921, paid an annual fee of £4 for each person registered after the Act. Nurses in the Dominions and other countries paid various yearly retention fees:

e.g. (1931) Australia—2s. 6d.
       Canada (Alberta) $4.00 (16s.)
       Various States of U.S.A.—50 c. to $2.00 (2s.–8s.)

In Scotland nurses had to return their certificates each year for endorsement, but of course the numbers were considerably smaller.

Over the next few years, approximately 2,000 names were removed annually for failure to pay the fee.

In 1936, pressure was brought to bear on the Council to reduce the fee and they finally agreed to do so, although the reduction from 2s. 6d. to 2s. caused a loss of revenue in the first year of over £2,000. As the numbers on the Register grew, this loss became proportionately greater; at the same time, the work required in sending reminders and compiling the Register increased. During the period under discussion the Council had to finance the new offices at 20 and 22 Portland Place—this was done by the sale of investments.

Balance sheets continued to show a reasonable margin most years but in 1937 a large amount of stock had to be sold to meet current expenditure.

The Finance Committee recommended to Council that they should become a participating Institution in the Federated Superannuation Scheme for nurses and hospital officers. By 1937 the Chairman was able to report that most of the office staff had joined the scheme.

THE TEST EXAMINATION

From 1929 onwards letters appeared in the nursing press on the need for some educational level of entry to nurse training. In 1932 the Council decided that after June 1936 no candidate could enter for the Preliminary State Examination who did not possess a General School Certificate or its equivalent, unless they passed an entrance examination set by the Council. This proposal met with considerable opposition from hospital managers who were afraid that it would cause a shortage of probationers and because of this they would have to employ more trained staff at higher salaries. In June 1935 the Minister was asked to approve the scheme with certain alterations: the resolution now read "that after June 1st, 1936, no candidate be admitted to a training school for the purposes of training for the State Examinations, who does not possess the General School Certificate or its equivalent, unless such candidates has passed, or passes within the trial period, a test examination in general education which will be set up by the General Nursing Council as an entrance examination; that the test examination take the form of a written examination of a simple type, with questions

THE GENERAL NURSING COUNCIL FOR ENGLAND AND WALES.

TEST EDUCATIONAL EXAMINATION.

ENGLISH AND GENERAL KNOWLEDGE.
(Time allowed 1½ hours)

**Question 1 is compulsory. The Candidate must
answer three out of the other four questions.**

1. Write for about half an hour on one of the following subjects :—
   (a) Description of a state or civic procession.
   (b) The difference Broadcasting has made to every-day life.
   (c) A description of the ideal house for four people (parents and two children).
   (d) An account of the one or two books you have most enjoyed during the last twelve months.
   (e) A description of an experiment you have seen or made.

2. Make use of each of the following words in a sentence, in such a way as to show that you
   understand its meaning :—
   > crisis, essential, ambassador, anticipate, temperature, temperament, conscious,
   > conscientious, credible, credulous.

3. (a) In what countries do the following people live : Esquimaux, Pygmies, Red Indians, Sikhs,
   Dutch ?
   (b) Name the authors of the following :—
   "David Copperfield," "Jane Eyre," "Vanity Fair," "Peter Pan," "The Jungle Book."
   (c) In what books do the following characters occur ? :—
   John Silver, the Mad Hatter, Titania, Minnehaha, Elizabeth Bennet.
   (d) Give the noun corresponding to each of the following adjectives :—
   real, visible, happy, true, transparent.

4. Complete the list below in the same way as in the examples given :—

(Lord Baldwin ... Statesman.	Sir Walter Scott ... Author.)
Marconi.	Shakespeare.
Pasteur.	Sir Malcolm Campbell.
Gainsborough.	Sir Ernest Shackleton.
Beethoven.	George Eliot.
Madame Curie.	Abraham Lincoln.

5. (a) Give the opposites of :—
   day, harmful, honest, misty, simple.

   (b) Fill in the missing words in the following quotations :—
   The quality of —— is not strained.
   To be or not to be, that is the ——.
   A fool and his —— are soon parted.
   Can the Ethiopian change his ——, or the —— his spots ?

   (c) In what cities are the following :—
   The Vatican, the Eiffel Tower, Fifth Avenue, Cleopatra's Needle, Holyrood ?

   (d) Re-write the following sentences, correcting where necessary :—
   Between you and I, the matter is hopeless.
   Do you want these letters posting ?
   Neither of them are here.
   If anyone has finished will they tell me ?
   This is the best of the two.

11. The first Test Educational Examination, 1937.
    (a) English and general knowledge.

THE GENERAL NURSING COUNCIL FOR ENGLAND AND WALES.

TEST EDUCATIONAL EXAMINATION.

The Candidate must attempt all questions set.

ARITHMETIC. $\frac{3}{4}$ hour.

[N.B.—All working must be shown.]

1. Add together : 4s. 7½d., 10s. 11d., 8s. 5¼d., 17s. 4½d.

2. Multiply 37·06 by 4·08.

3. Divide 18·3 by 12·45 correct to one decimal place.

4. Take the smallest of the following from the largest :—

$$\frac{17}{80}, \quad \frac{5}{16}, \quad \frac{2}{5}, \quad \frac{13}{120}.$$

5. A bottle contained 6 oz. of liquid ; half of it has been used, and I want to pour off 2 oz. What fraction of the liquid now in the bottle must I pour out ?

6. What is 6% of 25 galls. ? Express the answer in pints.

7. (a) Express 47 millimetres as centimetres.

   (b) Express ·52 grams as centigrams.

   (c) How many litres in 6,742 cubic centimetres ? (1 litre equals 1 cubic decimetre.)

8. In a certain home each bed must have a floor space of 100 sq. ft. and 1,000 cub. ft. of air. How many beds can you place in a room 80 ft. long, 32 ft. wide, and 20 ft. high ?

9. If a tea for 360 children costs £9, what will be the total cost if 100 more children come ?

10. Make a bill for the following :—

   6 sheets at 23s. 9d. a pair.
   12 pillow cases at 1s. 3d. each.
   22 tea cloths at 2½d. each.
   2 doz. yards of braid at 1¼d. a yard.
   Allow 5% discount for cash.

12. The first Test Educational Examination, 1937.

(b) Arithmetic.

on general knowledge, English and arithmetic: that if the recommendations are approved, a Board, in due course, be appointed to conduct the examination." The entrance fee was to be 5s.

Six months later (in January 1936) a letter was received from the Minister saying he would issue formal sanction of the test soon. In February, the Council received a letter from the London County Council saying that it had 10,000 nurses in its hospital service and stating its intention to ask the Minister to postpone his decision until its Council had submitted observations, since a detrimental effect on recruitment was feared. Miss Musson pointed out that the General Nursing Council's intentions had been made known in 1932, and so three and a half years' notice had been given. At the Council Meeting in November 1936 a letter from the Minister was read, in which he asked for a conference on the test and five members of the Council went to the Ministry for this.

In June 1937 a letter was received from the Minister agreeing the necessary changes in the Rules and Council wrote informing the training schools. The first test was held in November 1937; following this the papers were published in the nursing press and subsequently letters were received, some saying it was too hard and some too easy! Unfortunately, with the outbreak of hostilities in 1939 the test had to be abandoned "for the duration". In 1946 the Council attempted to re-establish an educational level of entry to training, but did not achieve this until 1962.

THE OFFICE AND STAFF

Some idea of the work in the office at this time can be given by the number of letters received and despatched:

1927—265,968 (exclusive of the election)
1928—285,000
1933—343,197

In 1932 the number of staff was over 50: there was at this time no difficulty in filling vacancies and it is interesting to note that in 1928 there were 77 applications for the post of Registration Officer.

The Minister had been informed, in 1927, that No. 20 Portland Place "would not be sufficient for the Council's needs for more than five years, if so long" and at the end of 1932, Council were advised to offer £15,000 for 22 Portland Place (next door to No. 20). Five rooms on the ground floor and the basement were immediately available and the sitting tenant would continue to rent the rest of the house. Some alterations were necessary.

The Council probably hoped that this would prove a permanent home, but at the beginning of 1935, they were approached by the British Broadcasting Corporation, and agreed to relinquish Nos. 20 and 22 Portland Place in exchange for the site of Nos. 23 and 25 and a sum adequate to cover the cost of a new building on a 999 years' lease, removal to the new premises, and compensation for loss of revenue.

Having achieved an extremely satisfactory bargain which gave them "purpose-built" offices for the first time, the Finance Committee felt able to recommend that £10,000 should be spent on the furnishings for the new building. During the negotiations, the B.B.C. and the Howard de Walden Estate gave permission for fittings such as Adam fireplaces and mahogany doors to be taken to the new offices. Also during the demolition of 23 and 25 Portland Place, certain Adam fittings and ceiling paintings thought to be by Cipriani were preserved and incorporated in the new building.

The exterior of the Council offices at 23 Portland Place is faced with Portland stone; the hall and main staircase are panelled with marble, and the stairs have margins of marble; all these conditions were stipulated by the Howard de Walden Estate. Building started in October 1935 and was completed by May 1937. The house consisted originally of a sub-basement, basement, ground floor and four upper floors, with provision in the structure for two further floors which were in fact added in 1961-62.

The hall

The fanlight over the entrance hall door was taken from the original No. 23, and that from No. 20 is incorporated in the glazed partition wall of one of the waiting rooms. Two antique mahogany chairs, bearing the crest of the Marquess of Winchester, stand in the hall. A fireplace from the demolished buildings has been fitted into the west wall of the hall; over the fireplace there is a plaque commemorating the opening of the new offices by Her Royal Highness the Princess Royal on Thursday, June 24th, 1937. Two ceiling paintings, one of Venus and one of Hermes have been inserted in the design of the hall ceiling.

The stair carpet which was specially woven, is of the same shade of blue as that used in the State Registration badge.

The first floor

Two ceiling paintings have been incorporated into the landing ceiling plaster—one of Diana and one of Bacchante; the iron ballustrading and mahogany doors were taken from the old premises.

The council room

This is on the front of the building and is 50 ft. long, 25 ft. wide and 16 ft. high. It is panelled in sycamore wood and there are seven ceiling paintings depicting Bacchus and Ariadne, Amorini, Hermes, a nymph at an altar, a Bacchanti, a flower offering and Ceres. There is a dais for the Chairman's desk and accompanying chairs, and in the well of the room are mahogany desks and leather upholstered chairs for members of Council. An anteroom to the Council room is also panelled in sycamore wood.

The cherry room is a room for smaller committee meetings to the right of the main staircase. This room is panelled in cherry wood and the rounded mantelpiece was preserved from the demolished building. There is a ceiling painting of Venus, the three Graces and Hera.

The table is the one which was used for Council meetings at 20 Portland Place.

The laurel room is to the left of the main staircase; it is panelled in Indian laurel wood and the ceiling paintings show Zeus and Ceres.

Next to the laurel room is the Chairman's room, panelled in English walnut; the furniture is also of walnut and the ceiling painting is of Venus and Cupid.

The blue room—so called owing to the colour of the leather upholstered furniture—is at the extreme west end of the first floor; it is used for large committee meetings. The ceiling painting is of Venus and Cupid and the walls are plaster. The refectory type mahogany table is 18 ft. long and the central design of the ceiling is reproduced in the veneer. The Chairman's chair in this room is the one used by the first Chairman of Council in 1920.

The Registrar's room, which is situated between the Chairman's room and the blue room, is panelled in Honduras cedar wood. The Seal of the Council is kept in this room and in this, and the three other rooms described, there are original Adam mantelpieces.

The other floors

The remainder of the rooms in the building are occupied by the administrative, executive and clerical staff of the Council. The basements are used for the storage of records, and the packing room. A multilith printing machine is also in the basement.

The opening ceremony

The Council met for the first time in its new premises on May 28th, 1937, but had to use the blue room as the furniture for the Council room had not arrived. The "move" had actually taken place on April 26th.

On June 24th, H.R. Highness arrived at 3 p.m. for the opening ceremony; visitors had been conducted to the Council chamber to await her. She was received by Miss Musson and the Mayor and Mayoress of St. Marylebone. A bouquet was presented by the Registrar.

Miss Musson in her speech of welcome told the story of the new building and gave details of the growth of the Council's work. Her Royal Highness declared the offices open; there was a prayer and blessing by the Bishop of Southwark, and Mr. Eason moved a vote of thanks. Among the guests who were presented were: Mrs. Fenwick, Mrs. Rowe, President of the College of Nursing; Miss Wilmshurst, General Superintendent of the Queen's Institute of District Nursing; Miss Riddell; members of Council; and the Vicar of All Souls Church, Langham Place.

Visitors saw among other things, the old manuscript Register, open at the first page. Tea was served on the fourth floor.

In the evening there was an informal party for 200–300 nurses and the office staff acted as guides.

EDUCATION AND EXAMINATIONS

The State examinations had continued since 1925 and one can estimate the progress of nurse training by giving some of the numbers of passes.

Final Examinations	General	Mental	Sick Children	Fever	Male
May 1929	1,157	24	53	140	1
May 1933	1,190	53	63	224	7

The failure rate varied overall, but the average for first entries was 20–30 per cent. Re-entries always had a much higher failure rate. It may be of interest to note that in May–June 1929, the total number passing the Final Examination in Scotland was 273, and in Northern Ireland was 36.

At the beginning of 1932 changes were made in fees to be paid to examiners: the cost in examiners' claims and subsistance was about £8,000 each time.

During 1933 the Education and Examination Committee revised the syllabus of examination and this was approved by the Minister; one object of this was to make the Preliminary Examination similar in all types of training.

During 1935 there was much discussion on the qualifications of lecturers. It was recommended that anatomy and physiology lectures should be given by recognised professors or lecturers in anatomy and physiology or by qualified practitioners who had held, at least, a resident post in hospital; revision classes were to be held by sister-tutors. Medical examiners were to be appointed for the oral examinations in anatomy and physiology and these were to be medical practitioners of good standing who had held a resident or other post on the staff of a hospital and who had had experience in teaching.

In 1937 a conference of the three statutory bodies for Great Britain and the Council for the Irish Free State was called to discuss this subject further.

In the period under discussion reciprocal registration was established with Victoria, Australia; the four states of South

Africa—Transvaal, Natal, Cape Province and Orange Free State; Tasmania; Burma; Madras; Southern Rhodesia; British Columbia; Manitoba; Alberta; and the territory for the seat of government, Canberra, Australia.

DISCIPLINE

In 1930 there was a report of the first prosecution actually instigated by the General Nursing Council: a nurse, who had falsely represented herself as State Registered, appeared in court and was fined £3. In the next two years, ten similar cases occurred.

In 1932 several letters were sent reprimanding nurses who had allowed their names to be used to advertise trade products and apologies were received.

In the five years 1928–32, seventeen names were removed from the Register and judgement was deferred in three cases. From 1933–7, twelve names were removed from the Register, and in six cases judgement was deferred. Twenty-six nurses were prosecuted during this period for falsely representing themselves as State Registered Nurses.

Reading the minutes and the press reports of the 1920s and 1930s one is forcibly struck by the public and professional attitude to those convicted of what, today, would be regarded as minor offences. On one occasion when a nurse, who had been convicted of shoplifting (a first offence) was not immediately struck off, scandalised letters appeared in the press about "keeping thieves on the Register". Two cases, in 1934 serve as an illustration; one nurse was struck off for staying in a hotel with a married man. Another nurse was struck off having been charged with misconduct; while the matron of a nursing home, she had a child whose father was employed on the staff: they subsequently married.

In 1933, in response to requests, Miss Musson published an article in the press, on the Council's procedure for disciplinary and penal cases as follows:

Investigation

(1) The name of the respondent is never published until a prima facie case has been established; this part is there-

fore taken in camera but the Council's solicitor is always present.

(2) If the case comes to the Council's notice after trial in court with a conviction but without imprisonment, the Council

(a) decides if a prima facie case had been made;

(b) gives the respondent an opportunity to attend and give evidence. If a prison sentence has been given the Council may, forthwith and without further enquiry, remove the name of the nurse from the Register.

(3) If the case is not tried in court, Council must prove the charges to be true before taking action.

(4) The respondent is always informed of the charge, by registered post, and given due notice of the date the case will come before Council. She may appear and may be represented by a solicitor, or friends. The case must be proved before evidence of character is given.

Procedure

The Chairman asks the Council's solicitor to state the case: only relevant evidence is given. Witnesses are called, if necessary. The respondent (or representative) may cross-examine and give evidence. Members of Council can cross-examine through the Chairman or solicitor. If the charge is proved, the respondent, or friend, or representative may produce extenuating circumstances, evidence of good character, etc.

The Council deliberates in camera; the respondent and others are recalled to hear the decision.

The decision may be:

(1) Removal of the respondent's name from the Register: in this case the respondent receives a copy of the Rules with the procedure for application for restoration at a later date.

(2) Removal of the respondent's name for a period. In this case, at the end of the prescribed period the nurse's name is automatically restored without evidence of good character. (At the time of writing this article this had never been done.)

(3) Sentence postponed; this is similar to probation and the respondent has to produce evidence of good character at the end of a specified time.

PERSONALITIES

Miss Musson continued as Chairman from 1928–38 and in May 1932 she went to Leeds to receive an honorary Doctorate of Laws from the University. At the next Council meeting, in answer to congratulations she said "the honour was far beyond her deserts, nevertheless it was a wonderfully generous mark of encouragement to the nursing profession . . . and to the work of the Council . . . a very high compliment to the work of those who fought for so many years to obtain State Registration".

Miss Cox-Davies was vice-Chairman in 1929, 1930, 1931, 1933, 1934, and 1938; Miss Sparshott in 1932, and Miss Darbyshire from 1935–7.

In 1934, Miss Alicia Lloyd Still had the D.B.E. conferred upon her in the Birthday Honours and received the congratulations of the Council.

During this decade, several people who played an outstanding part either in the fight for registration, or in the early days of the Council, died. They included Lady Hobhouse (1927), Rev. G. B. Cronshaw (1928), Sir Jenner Verrall (1929), Sir Richard Barnett (1930), Lord Knutsford (1931), Dr. Bedford Pierce (1932), Mr. Sidney Pitt, solicitor to the Council (1935), and Sir Wilmot Herringham and Mr. West, the Council's auditor (in 1936). Mr. Hewitt Pitt succeeded his father as the Council's solicitor in 1933.

In 1929, Miss Musson and Miss Cox-Davies represented the General Nursing Council at the International Congress of Nurses in Montreal. (In their absence, Miss Sparshott acted as Chairman, and Miss Hogg as vice-Chairman.) They took with them exhibits of the Council's work, which were shown on a stand at Montreal; these included the current Register, replicas of the State Registered badge and certificate and a doll dressed in the official registered uniform. When the I.C.N. Congress was held in London in 1937, Council members and staff were able to have useful meetings with representatives of Registration bodies in the dominions.

In March 1929, the Council held its 100th meeting. Four members, at that time, had been present since its inception; they were Miss Cox-Davies who had attended 92 meetings; Miss Villiers, 89; Miss Lloyd-Still, 85; and Miss Sparshott, 69 meetings. The 500th Council meeting will be held during the Jubilee year.

In 1937, 400 seats on the Coronation route were allocated to the profession by the Ministry of Health and these were distributed via the General Nursing Council.

In January 1937, comments on the forthcoming election began to appear in the press. One quoted the London Branch of the College of Nursing as pointing out that the personnel of the College Council should be entirely different from that of the General Nursing Council. "Many outside authorities have found it difficult to regard an opinion by either as entirely independent of each other, when they are aware that many members serve on both Councils"[10].

In April, the Finance Committee agreed to approve the sum of £231 15s. 2d. for stationery for the election.

In September, the press said that some of the issues this time were the re-organisation of the three or four years "general training"—this referred to a suggestion for a comprehensive training and the enrolment, or control, of assistant nurses.

A change was seen in the College of Nursing policy, in that they decided not to join with other organisations in preparing their list of recommended candidates. They said that only those who had time to perform the arduous duties required should be nominated.

Returning to an earlier theme, an article in the press, in October, said that it was no wonder nurses did not know the difference between the College and the General Nursing Council since eight of the existing eleven elected "general" nurses on the latter also served on the College Council; these were Miss Cox-Davies, Miss Dey, Miss Gullan, Miss Innes, Miss Jones, Dame Alicia, Miss Musson and Miss Sparshott[11].

Fifty candidates stood for the sixteen seats—a record number: of these, 36 were candidates for the eleven general seats, five for the male nurses' representative, five for the two mental nurses' seats, three for the sick children's nurses' representative, and the fever nurses' candidate was unopposed. At a meeting in the Cowdray Hall in November, the College nominated their twelve candidates.

The election was held in December 1937 with the following result:

Elected

General seats	*Votes*	
New members:		
Miss G. M. Bowes	8,242	Matron, Birmingham Hospital Centre
Miss A. Burgess	8,368	Matron, Crumpsall Hospital, Manchester
Miss L. G. Duff Grant	9,098	Lady Superintendent, Manchester Royal Infirmary
Miss M. Milne	8,878	Matron, Bolingbroke Hospital, London
Miss E. Pearce	12,360	Sister-Tutor, Middlesex Hospital, London
Miss D. M. Smith	9,070	Matron, Middlesex Hospital, London
Re-elected:		
Miss R. A. Cox-Davies	10,078	
Miss H. Dey	9,779	
Miss M. Jones	8,552	
Miss E. E. P. Mac-Manus	12,745	
Miss E. M. Musson	9,686	
Male nurse (new):		
Mr. R. J. Ousby	74	Charge Nurse, Walton Hospital, Liverpool
Mental nurses:		
Miss K. M. Willis	1,428	re-elected
Mr. J. H. Buckley	1,653	re-elected
Sick Children's nurse (new):		
Miss D. A. Lane	639	Matron, The Hospital for Sick Children, Gt. Ormond Street, London.
Fever (new):		
Miss F. M. Campbell	—	S.E. Fever Hospital, London, unopposed

Appointed

Board of Education:	Miss Gwatkin, re-appointed
	Miss M. E. Edwards
Privy Council:	Sir Henry Gooch, B.A., LL.B., J.P., Governor of St. Bartholomew's Hospital and King's College Hospital
	Countess of Limerick, re-appointed
Ministry of Health:	Dr. Geoffrey Evans, M.A., M.D., F.R.C.P., M.R.C.S., St. Bartholomew's Hospital
	Sir Frederick Menzies, K.B.E., M.D., LL.D., Medical Officer of Health, L.C.C.
	Miss Puxley, O.B.E., Principal, Ministry of Health
	Dr. Collins ⎱ re-appointed Dr. Kettle ⎰

The returning officer gave the following figures. The electorate was 86,734; but as there was only one fever candidate, only 79,986 voting papers were issued. 32,660 valid votes were received (approximately 41 per cent); the voting papers had filled 166 mail bags and weighed nearly two tons. The percentage of the electorate who voted was higher than at the previous election, but unfortunately "in 126 papers (folded while the ink still wet) it was quite impossible to decide which marks were votes and which blots".

References

1. *Nursing Times*—23.6.28.
2. *British Journal of Nursing*—September 1928.
3. *Nursing Times*—3.11.28.
4. *British Journal of Nursing*—December 1928.
5. Ibid.—September 1930.
6. Ibid.—July 1932.
7. *Nursing Times*—1.10.32.
8. Ibid.—26.11.32.
9. Ibid.—3.2.34.
10. Ibid.—9.1.37.
11. Ibid,—9,10,37,

Chapter 7

THE WAR YEARS

"The maxim of the British people is, 'business as usual'."
WINSTON CHURCHILL

Towards the end of 1938, the growing fear of impending war concentrated everyone's attention on the need for planning in case of a national emergency. The Government set up two committees for England and Wales, a Nursing Emergency Committee and a Medical Emergency Committee.

The Central Emergency Committee for the Nursing Profession for civilian defence in time of emergency, was to:

(1) ascertain the nurse power of the country (with the assistance of the *Royal College of Nursing); and

(2) compile a register of nursing auxiliaries who were prepared to offer their services in an emergency (through the Order of St. John and the British Red Cross Society).

The committee was to be supervised by the Ministry of Health and was to work closely with hospital authorities, the Order of St. John and the British Red Cross Society.

Those familiar with the composition of committees today will not be surprised to learn that, although the Medical Committee consisted solely of doctors and departmental representatives, the Nursing Committee consisted of the following: eleven men representing doctors, hospital administrators and local and central government officials and nine women of whom only five were nurses—the Matrons-in-Chief of the three Services, and one representative each of the Royal College of Nursing and the General Nursing Council. The latter's nominee to the Committee was †Dame Ellen Musson, who asked that Miss Cox-Davies should be allowed to deputise for her when necessary[1].

The General Nursing Council was only too aware that an emergency would effect all aspects of its work. At the Council meeting on May 26th, 1939, Miss Gwatkin moved and Miss Cox-Davies seconded, "that in the event of National emergency the Chairman of Council and/or the Vice-Chairman and/or the

* The College of Nursing was granted a Charter in 1928 and permission to use the title 'Royal' was given in 1939.
† Miss Musson was made D.B.E. in 1939.

Chairman of any standing committee, be authorised to act for the Council and to take such steps as may appear necessary to carry on the work of the Council". This resolution was forwarded to the Minister, and at the Council meeting in July, his reply was read; it stated that he had no power to sanction departures from the Rules which had been approved by him. He suggested that the Council should draft the necessary amendments to the Rules which could be put in cold storage in case a state of emergency arose, when they could be put before both Houses of Parliament.

Two amendments were drafted and approved by Council:
(1) To discontinue the Test Examination if this were thought to be desirable;
(2) To vest power in the Chairman, Vice-Chairman and Chairman of a standing committee.

In October, after the declaration of war, these amendments were approved.

In September, October, November and December 1939 there were no meetings of the full Council. Routine business was carried on by a committee composed of Dame Ellen, Chairman of Council; Miss D. Smith, Vice-Chairman of Council and Chairman of the Registration Committee; Mr. Buckley, Chairman of the Mental Nurses Committee; Miss Cox-Davies, Chairman of the General Purposes Committee; Miss Dey, Chairman of the Education and Examinations Committee; Miss Gwatkin, Chairman of the Finance Committee; and Miss Jones, Chairman of the Disciplinary Committee.

Three specific points were discussed during this time.

It had been hoped that the Minister would allow the Council to waive the payment of the annual retention fee for those nurses in difficulty due to the war; but this proved impossible as the Council had no power, under the Act, to suspend payment.

At a meeting with representatives of the British Red Cross Society, St. John Ambulance Association and the Central Emergency Committee, the position of V.A.D.s and Civil Nursing Auxiliaries, who wished to train as nurses, was discussed. The Council's representatives stated that there could be no reduction in training.

Some of the rules regarding nurse-training within one hospital were discussed and relaxed, since it was obvious that movement of student nurses would take place.

In January 1940, the full Council met, and heard that the Central Committee for Nursing was to cease to function at the end of the month; it was to be superseded by the Civil Nursing Reserve Advisory Council, and the General Nursing Council's nominee to this was Miss D. M. Smith, the Vice-Chairman.

TRAINING AND EXAMINATIONS

At the outbreak of the war, the Government drew up plans for the hospital service and divided England and Wales into regions and sectors. In addition, hospitals in industrial and heavily populated areas made plans, where necessary, to evacuate patients and some of the staff, to premises in less vulnerable areas. This obviously called for re-arrangements in the system of examinations and training and in September 1939, the Council issued a statement:

Training

London: The following arrangements will apply in the case of the hospitals in the ten London Sectors, viz.: that in each sector of the London area, all the hospitals—general, children's, fever, mental and mental defectives hospitals— will be considered as one hospital in each category, for the purposes of the training of nurses.

Provinces: The following arrangements will apply in the case of hospitals in any industrial area where decentralisation of hospitals is ordered, viz.: that in each region serving a decentralised area, all the hospitals—general, children's, fever, mental and mental defectives hospitals—will be considered as one hospital in each category for the purposes of the training of nurses.

Examinations

1. Written examinations and marking of papers:

These examinations will be held in each hospital where there are candidates, and the answers despatched by the presiding examiners direct to the examiners marking the books in the sector or region. The examiners results should be made in duplicate, one set sent to Headquarters, and the other set kept in a safe place.

2. Oral and practical examinations:
  (i) These will be held in each hospital where there are candidates.
  (ii) The rule requiring that candidates should not be examined by examiners from their own training school, will be waived.
  (iii) The group of examiners for the Preliminary State Examination will be composed of one medical practitioner and one nurse examiner; the nurse examiner will be asked to include one question on hygiene.
  (iv) The group of examiners for the Final State Examination will be composed of a physician, a surgeon and a nurse.

Other details of changes included the following:

The written examination was reduced by half an hour on each paper.

The written examination could start an hour before the stated time; if there was a large enough group of candidates, half could start at 8.0 a.m. and the second half at 10.0 a.m., provided the two sets did not meet.

In cases of difficulty, the matron could arrange substitute examiners for the oral and practical parts of the examination.

The statement ended by saying that the Test Educational Examination was discontinued for the time being; the Registrar had been given power to return the fee paid for cancelled Test Examinations.

Specific arrangements were made for those male student nurses called up for military service. These included allowing those who had made arrangements for, but had not yet taken, the Test, to be exempt on return to training, and allowing those whose training was interrupted by military service to return, with no additional period required for the break in training.

As conditions in the hospitals were changing every day during the first few months of the war, and as the Council needed time to make alternative arrangements, the October 1939 State Examinations were cancelled; they were held during November and December 1939 and in some cases continued into January 1940. This inevitably led to a delay in the February Examinations which eventually took place in April 1940. The rules were altered so that any student nurse who would have completed one year of training by May 14th, could take the Preliminary

Examination in April, provided the lectures had been completed. A similar provision was made for Final candidates whose training would be completed by May 30th.

In May 1940 attention was drawn by an article in the press to the effect that war-time conditions were having on nurses and nurse training. This highlighted the problems due to evacuation, periods of inactivity, poor equipment in emergency hospitals, lack of some experience and living in billets instead of nurses homes[2]. This theme was developed in November 1940 by a leader on "continuing training". It pointed out that evacuation "has so changed the scope of work available in many hospitals as to make them no longer suitable to be used as training schools"[3]. In the large cities, sector matrons could transfer students from one hospital to another of the same type to ensure adequate experience, but in the small towns this was obviously more difficult.

At the October Council meeting (1940) it was reported that the latest examination "had gone off fairly well, although orals and practicals in London had had to be postponed because of air raids". Dame Ellen said there had been difficulties, but she was sure the Council would be very grateful to all who had helped to overcome them. For instance, in one big provincial city the question papers arrived five days after the examinations, but the Matron had sent off to another centre for a paper and chalked the questions on a blackboard. At one London centre the desks failed to arrive, so the candidates sat on the floor and used their chairs as desks. This made the use of ink difficult so candidates were given indelible pencils.

After a year of difficulties the Council obviously felt that it was in everyones interest to hold the examinations twice yearly instead of three times: "and to permit candidates to enter for the examination preceding the first examination for which they would have been entitled to enter". With these arrangements, about 200 written centres and 400 oral and practical centres were needed, half for the Preliminary and half for the Final Examinations. The dates were to be in early April and late September. The number of candidates involved was about 8,000 each time for the Preliminary and 5,000 for the Final Examination. More time was also allowed for the return of entrance forms.

In March 1942 the Council approved that arrangements be made through the Prisoner of War Department and through the External Department of the University of London, "to enable Prisoners of War to enter for the written part of Part 1 of the Preliminary Examination, and that no fee be charged. If however the candidate, at a later date, is in a position to complete the Preliminary Examination the fees for the whole examination will be payable". Later in the year the Council ran into difficulties over another proposal: it was decided to "refuse to admit, to any of the Council's examinations, even candidates who had completed their studies, without being under any obligation to state their reason". The G.N.C. felt they were acting in the candidates best interests since information from the police might be involved and the Council's solicitor had himself suggested the wording; however the Bristol Branch of the Royal College of Nursing felt the decision was "unnecessarily arbitrary". In October, November and December 1942, questions were asked about the wording of the proposal in the House of Commons and Mr. Ernest Brown (the Minister) said: "I am making enquiries". In January 1943 the proposed Rule was altered to read "Should it come to the notice of the Council that a candidate for entrance to any of the Council's Examinations had been convicted of a felony or misdemeanour, or had been guilty of conduct which, had she been a Registered Nurse, would, in the opinion of the Council, have rendered her liable to disciplinary action under the Rules of the Council and the removal of her name from the Register, the Council may, after giving the candidate an opportunity of stating her case and making other reasonable investigations as may be necessary, refuse to admit her to the examination in question". The Minister signed the Rule five weeks later.

Pre-nursing courses

It will be remembered that the first time that candidates from pre-nursing courses took Part 1 of the Preliminary Examination was in December 1939. In February 1940 the Board of Education invited the G.N.C. to discuss the question of relaxing the regulations for pre-nursing courses. As a war-time measure the Council agreed to accept teachers with a degree in biology or zoology to teach anatomy and physiology in pre-nursing courses. By October 1940, 30 one-year courses were approved and this number continued to grow to reach 199 by 1944.

Comprehensive schemes of training

During the war years more interest was shown in the possibility of establishing four-year comprehensive schemes of training. A sub-committee of the Education and Examinations Committee was set up to consider the possibility; the conclusions reached were that there should be a four-year course with:

(1) An 8–12 weeks' Preliminary Training School.

(2) At least two years in the parent hospital, to cover general medicine and surgery and pass the Preliminary Examination before secondment (two members disagreed with this).

(3) The basic course was to include:

Medicine: 3 months each male and female.
Surgery: 3 months each male and female.
Gynaecology: 2 months.
Paediatrics: 2 months.
Out patient department/Casualty: 1–2 months.
Theatre: 1–2 months.

(4) In addition:

Fevers: 3 months
and experience in orthopaedics
,,   obstetrics
,,   ear, nose and throat
,,   skins
,,   eyes
,,   V.D.

The sub-committee felt that while the sick children and mental registers should remain, the fever training might at some time come to an end. It is obvious from the records that several of the seven members of the sub-committee had divergent views on comprehensive training, and possibly because of this no real progress was made. However, it was decided to hold a conference on this and on revision of the various syllabuses in 1945.

Special training

In 1943 the shortage of nurses in sanatoria and other special hospitals led to a statement by the G.N.C. that it regarded this type of experience as of great value to a nurse, and drew attention to the existing arrangements for such experience:

(1) The Council permitted nurses in training in complete general hospitals to be seconded to sanatoria for a period not exceeding three months.

(2) Schemes of affiliation might be arranged between general and special hospitals, including sanatoria. This normally meant two years' experience in the special hospital, culminating in the Preliminary Examination, followed by two years' experience in the general hospital.

(3) The Council was prepared to consider schemes which afforded comprehensive training, provided they included not less than two years in a complete general training school.

The position in the special hospitals must have been especially difficult during the war years since most people, while recognising the need for service, preferred to work in either the larger general hospitals or the forces. The Council in fact drew up Rules for post-registration training and examinations for tuberculosis, and orthopaedic nurses and these were mentioned in the Chairman's report in 1944.

During the war approval of training schools continued, a limited number of inspections were carried out and all the syllabuses of subjects for examination were revised.

FINANCE

In March 1939 the Council took stock of its financial affairs. During the previous year they had a deficit of £3,000 which would have been £6,000 had not stock been sold at a profit. Council discussed the question of the examination fees and whether these should be raised, since it was felt they were rather lower than those of similar bodies. The Chairman pointed out that if capital were exhausted, the fees would have to be raised a great deal; also that one guinea of the Final Examination fee was looked on as a Registration fee, and taking this into account, the Registration Department was self supporting. Seventeen members agreed that the fee should be raised, but four were against. When the situation was pointed out to the Minister he asked if the Council could not effect economies.

Although the reduction of sixpence in the annual retention fee had seemed a small one in 1936, it resulted in an annual loss to the Council of from £2,000–£3,000 and the accounts had shown a deficit since the date of its institution. This subject was under discussion for some time and in July 1943 the Minister was asked to sanction:

(a) that a charge of two shillings and sixpence be made for the original Registration certificate,

(b) a reversion to two shillings and sixpence for the annual retention fee, and

(c) that a charge of one shilling be made for a uniform permit.

The deficit for the year ending March 31st, 1942 had been met from the General Purposes fund, but Council realised that in future the deficit would be much greater. The 1943 Nurses Act extended the Council's responsibilities to the training and enrolment of assistant nurses and as this involved setting up a completely new department, which would not be self-supporting for some time, costs were bound to rise.

The Minister wanted more information before agreeing to raise the retention fee, and the British College of Nurses expressed strong dissatisfaction at the idea of raising the retention fee of registered nurses to finance the enrolment of assistant nurses. Dame Ellen pointed out that the pre-war fee of two shillings no longer covered war time costs, and the Minister finally agreed to the increase from January 20th, 1944; this was to be in respect of the fee payable for the retention of a name on the Register for 1945.

With regard to the costs of the assistant nurses the Minister would not ask the Treasury for a loan in view of the Council's large reserves and suggested they should meet their expenses by an overdraft from the bank.

During the war, Council continued to pay superannuation contributions for nurse members of its staff released for war service.

In 1944 the estimates for the forthcoming election expenses were £669 16s. 9d. for stationery (£231 15s. 2d. in 1937) and £1,468 6s. 4d. for printing.

By the end of the war the salaries of the Council's staff totalled £1,000 per week.

ASSISTANT NURSES

In the later months of 1933 and the first part of 1934, references can be found in the nursing press to the need for "assistant nurses". At the time, the need was linked to the economic depression since the trained nurse had to be paid a considerably higher salary than the untrained helper—especially for the care of the sick at home.

The matter was discussed at the annual conference of the College of Nursing and one speaker stated that there was a need for trained orderlies, with a two-year training up to the Preliminary Examination standard, to provide stable staff. At the April (1934) meeting of the General Nursing Council, a letter was read from Miss Wilmshurst, General Superintendent of the Queens' Institute of District Nurses; she stressed the problem of unemployment and pointed out that more probationers were being trained than could find employment when they were registered. She felt that the Council should take steps to ensure a reduction in the numbers being trained and should consider withdrawing approval from some of the smaller, affiliated hospitals. In reply, the Council pointed out that, under the Act, it had no power to limit the number of candidates, and if a small hospital could provide the necessary training, approval could not be withdrawn.

In some areas practical steps were taken to provide assistant nurses; the Local Authorities in Essex realised that nursing standards in some hospitals were not all they should be, and since they had difficulty in staffing hospitals for the chronic and infirm, they instituted what soon became known as the Essex scheme. The County Supervisor of Nursing, Miss Snowden, worked out and initiated, a two-year training scheme for young women with no nursing experience and submitted details to the Ministry of Health. The Ministry said it was a matter for the General Nursing Council, but the latter had to point out that, under the Act, such women could not be recognised as nurses since a three-year training was specified.

At a conference held in 1935 the scheme was discussed; speakers were obviously concerned, not only that a second grade of nurse was being created, but also that in the current economic circumstances employing authorities might deliberately choose to employ the "cheaper" grade. Miss Musson made it clear that the General Nursing Council neither approved nor disapproved—it simply had no statutory power in this respect. It was obvious that the Essex scheme was working well and had 67 such nurses.

The whole subject was a "talking point" and another meeting was held in the Cowdray Hall, by the College of Nursing in October 1936, on "the second grade of nurse". The meeting was held in response to a letter from Miss Musson to the College Council, asking whether they were in favour of a special grade of nurse for the chronic sick, and if so, under what authority the training should be carried out. It was pointed out that the letter was a personal one, and was not written in Miss Musson's capacity as Chairman of the General Nursing Council. At the meeting the chair was taken by Miss D. M. Smith and at the end a vote was taken; 56 of those present wanted a special grade and 30 were against; 53 wanted the General Nursing Council to be responsible for training and one felt it should be in the hands of municipal bodies. The editorial comment in the *Nursing Times* was, "what chance has a register for nurses for the chronic sick? Considerable pressure has failed to establish a register for tuberculosis nursing"[4].

Two months later, the elected members of the General Nursing Council met representatives of the nursing organisations to discuss a second grade of nurse; one of the representatives said that an approved "Roll" was needed.

In February 1937, the Professional Association Committee of the College of Nursing passed a recommendation that "the College ask the General Nursing Council for guidance as to the establishment of a Roll of trained special workers to carry out the domestic nursing duties in the wards of chronic institutions and amongst the community". Miss Musson stated that, first the General Nursing Council was not an advisory body, and second the Minister of Health had advised that under the Act the Council had no power to act in this matter. Miss Rundle, General Secretary of the College, asked whether the Act could be amended and if not whether the College should ask the Minister how such a Roll could be set up. Miss Musson said there was no unanimity amongst the nurses' organisations as to the need for a second grade of nurse; such a grave step should not be hurried. It was not as though the chronic sick were not being nursed at all, since assistant nurses were doing this work all the time[5].

On reading the literature of this time one gets the impression of frequent discussion and correspondence between two independent bodies, but one must remember (see page 117) that of the eleven elected general nurses on the General Nursing Council, eight also served on the College Council.

In November 1937, an Inter-Departmental Committee on Nursing Services was established to report to the Minister of Health and the President of the Board of Education; the terms of reference included inquiries into . . . recruitment, training and registration and terms and conditions of service of persons engaged in nursing the sick. Although no final report was ever published, due to the outbreak of war, an interim report was produced, dated December 1938. The chairman was the Earl of Athlone and there were twenty members, four of whom were nurses; one of these was Miss Musson. The Committee recommended that the grade of nurse known as the assistant nurse should be given a recognised status and placed on a Roll under the control of the General Nursing Council.

In February 1939, the Royal British Nurses' Association and the British College of Nurses wrote to the Council protesting against the formation of a Roll.

At the Council meeting in May 1939, a letter was received from the Minister asking for observations on the formation of a Roll of assistant nurses. The Council replied that the matter had already been considered and was approved, on condition that the legislation envisaged was implemented before the Roll was established.

The outbreak of war focused attention on other more urgent matters for some time, and also introduced large numbers of auxiliary workers into many hospitals. However in 1941, the Royal College of Nursing set up a large committee under the chairmanship of Lord Horder—the Nursing Reconstruction Committee; its terms of reference were "to consider ways and means of implementing the recommendations of the Inter-Departmental Committee on Nursing Services". The Committee's report was prepared and issued in four sections—the whole over a period of seven years. Section 1, on the assistant nurse, was published in 1942. Its recommendations included:

(i) that the term assistant nurse be adhered to;

(ii) that the assistant nurse be enrolled under the control of the General Nursing Council;

(iii) suggestions as to the qualification for admission to the Roll, for existing, intermediate and future assistant nurses;

(iv) that training should be for two years and that student nurses (training for the Register) and pupil nurses (training for the Roll) should be trained in separate hospitals, or separate parts of the same hospital.

The Committee felt that "the position of the assistant nurse is pivotal. Far from lacking importance, the assistant nurse of the future, as envisaged by the Committee, should become one of the most stable elements in our national nursing services—an integral part of the profession and a person whose status offers the key to the improved training of her senior partner, the State Registered nurse"[6].

In 1943, a Bill was introduced into the House of Commons to provide, amongst other things, "for the enrolment of assistant nurses for the sick.

The 1943 Nurses Act

This was the first piece of new legislation affecting the statutory body and nurse training to come into force since 1919 —twenty-four years before; it is interesting that in the twenty-four years following 1943 there have been five Acts and numerous Orders and Amendments to Rules.

The 1943 Act had three parts dealing with:

(1) The enrolment of assistant nurses;

(2) Agencies for the supply of nurses;

(3) Miscellaneous and general points, including matters relating to teachers of nursing, penalties for false representation as a nurse, and the opening of the list of certain nurses not registered or enrolled.

In Part 1 of the Act, there were six sections, dealing with the Roll itself, the Rules, the Assistant Nurses Committee, the right of appeal in disciplinary matters and over approval of training schools, and the restriction of the use of the title nurse and assistant nurse.

The similarity between the 1919 and the 1943 Acts is striking both in their length and content. Section 1 stated that "it shall be the duty of the General Nursing Council for England and Wales to form and keep a Roll of assistant nurses subject to and in accordance with the provisions of this Act"[7].

Section 2 said that the Council were to make Rules:

(a) for regulating the formation, maintenance and publication of the Roll;

(b) for regulating the conditions of admission to the Roll;

(c) for regulating the conduct of examinations;

(d) relating to the removal of and restoration of names to the Roll;

(e) making provision for certificates, uniform and badge.

The Rules had to lay down the prescribed training, details of approval of training schools and conditions for the enrolment of existing assistant nurses.

Existing assistant nurses were to be admitted to the Roll "on producing evidence to the satisfaction of the Council that they are of good character, are of the prescribed age, are persons who were for at least the prescribed period before the seventeenth day of March, 1943, bona fide engaged in practice as nurses under conditions which appear to the Council to be satisfactory for the purposes of this provision and have such knowledge and experience of nursing as to justify their enrolment"[8].

Section 3 said that the Assistant Nurses Committee was to be constituted in accordance with the provisions contained in the first Schedule to the Act. There were to be eleven members: six appointed by the Council and five to represent assistant nurses. Those appointed by the Council were to come from its own membership, but one was not to be a registered nurse. For the first Committee, the representatives of assistant nurses were to be appointed by the Minister, but once the Roll was established, four were to be elected by enrolled nurses and one appointed by the Minister. The term of office of the first Committee was to be three years and after that, five years.

The power and duties of the Assistant Nurses Committee were clearly defined and limited. They were to consider any matter which wholly or mainly concerned assistant nurses and to report on it to the Council, who would receive and consider the report before taking action. The only matters in which the

Committee had statutory authority were disciplinary matters relating to enrolled nurses and "any other matter referred to the Committee in so far as the Council expressly authorise the Committee to deal with it"[9].

Section 4 laid down the fee to be paid by existing assistant nurses as one guinea; all enrolled assistant nurses were to pay an annual retention fee not exceeding two shillings and sixpence.

When the General Nursing Council discussed the Bill, it was noted that the new regulations had to be laid before each House for 40 days—this period had previously been 21 days.

Mrs. Fenwick—now an old lady of 86—was horrified at the prospect of a second grade of nurse and spent much time at the House of Commons attempting to lobby Members of Parliament to persuade them to vote against the Bill; she was present in the House at all three readings. It was finally passed on Wednesday, April 7th, 1943; a number of nurses attended the debate and they were struck by the very small number of Members present[10].

In 1905, recommendation 21 of the Select Committee on the Registration of Nurses had suggested that once a General Nursing Council was set up, it should within four years, report to the Privy Council "on the desirability of a separate register of nurses whose training is of a lower standard than that laid down for the Register of Nurses"[11]. It had taken 24 years, and Mrs. Fenwick had opposed it throughout.

The Assistant Nurses Committee

The members of the Assistant Nurses Committee were announced at the Council meeting in May 1943. Those appointed by the Minister of Health were:

Miss R. Dreyer. Public Health Department, London County Council.

Miss L. Snowden. Lady Supervisor of Nurses, Essex County Council.

Mrs. W. L. Forde. Matron, Wordsley Emergency Hospital, Stourbridge, Worcs.

Mrs. Henry Brooke. Member of Council, Queens Institute of District Nurses and wife of an M.P.

Miss Elizabeth Tracey, an assistant nurse from Derby.

Dame Ellen and Miss Smith drew up a suggested list of nominees which was unanimously approved by the Council; they were:

> Dame Ellen Musson
> Miss D. M. Smith
> Miss A. Burgess
> Miss F. M. Campbell
> Dr. H. M. C. Macaulay
> Miss E. Pearce

It was also announced that "the historic first meeting of the Assistant Nurses Committee will take place on June 11th".

At the July Council meeting, the Chairman of the Committee, Dr. Macaulay, presented its report; it contained the draft Rules for existing and intermediate assistant nurses, which were discussed in camera, and were submitted to the Minister. When they were published, the Rules were extremely reminiscent of those drawn up for the State Register—with one striking difference. In the 1919 Act, the words "shall in any case be a female" appeared; in the new Rules for the Roll, the phrase was "the feminine gender includes the masculine". The *Nursing Times* pointed out the anomaly that whereas male nurses had a special part of the Register, there was only one Roll for both men and women[12]. The Council had approached the Minister on this point, but he had stated that any alteration to the Register would need an Amendment to the 1919 Act and this had not been proposed.

The Rules for existing nurses during the two-year period of grace were as follows:

in order to enroll, an existing nurse had to produce evidence of two years' whole-time training, or experience under the supervision of trained nursing staff, in a hospital or institution, before March 17th, 1943;

or three years' whole-time practice in sick nursing, with six months' training, or experience under the supervision of trained nursing staff in a hospital or institution;

or—for State Certified Midwives—evidence of three years' nursing the sick and/or midwifery, including not less than six months' training, or experience in a hospital or institution (this was to cover the village nurse/midwives);

or evidence of five years' whole-time bona fide practice in nursing the sick before March 17th, 1943, including such recent experience as the Council considered adequate. Applicants in this last category had to produce the names of three referees, one registered nurse and two doctors, to give evidence of character, competence, knowledge and experience. No applicants could be under 20 years of age and all had to submit a birth certificate.

Rules were made for those (intermediate assistant nurses) who would finish training after March 17th, 1943, and before the new examination system came into being; they had to produce evidence of two years' whole-time training, or experience under the supervision of trained nursing staff, one year of which must have been spent in one hospital or institution, or in hospitals under one authority, unless the Council decided otherwise; or evidence that before January 1st, 1947, the applicant had become a State Certified Midwife and had had the specified training.

In January 1944, the Minister stated that he had no objection to the appointment of salaried inspectors for assistant nurses centres of instruction, but said that the Council must bear the cost. The G.N.C.'s comment was that it had never been able to afford this for student nurses.

At the Council meeting in February 1944, two recommendations from the Assistant Nurses Committee were approved:

(i) that the Roll of Assistant Nurses be opened on March 20th, 1944 and that an official notice announcing this be sent to the press;

(ii) that two inspectors of training schools for assistant nurses be appointed, who shall be State Registered Nurses, having experience as ward sisters, in hospital administration and in the training of nurses. The appointment in the first instance is to be on a temporary basis at a commencing salary of £425 per annum, plus travelling and subsistence allowance.

It was also announced that the Minister had approved the Rules for existing and intermediate assistant nurses.

By May 1944 the draft syllabus of training was ready, was circulated to appropriate bodies and was finally sent to the Minister.

The syllabus of training was published in 1945 and formed the 5th Schedule to the Rules framed under Part 1, Section 2 of the Nurses Act 1943.

The syllabus stated that all subjects were to be taught in a simple and essentially practical manner.

There were six parts:

Part 1—Introduction which included nursing and its place in the community.
Personal qualities required in a nurse and responsibilities to patients and property.
Patients in hospital.
The hospital as a unit.

Part 2—Body structure and functions in health.
Elementary hygiene.
The laws of healthy living.
The maintenance of health.

Part 3—First Aid.

Part 4—General Nursing. Care of patients.
Routine nursing procedures.
Handling of equipment.

Part 5—The nursing duties and attention required during illness.
The main features of disease.

Part 6—(Applicable only to those pupils who spent part of
A   the period of training in a hospital or sanitorium for the treatment of pulmonary tuberculosis.)
Nursing and care of patients suffering from pulmonary tuberculosis.

B   (Applicable only to those pupils who spent part of the period of training in an infectious disease hospital.)
Nursing and care of patients suffering from infectious diseases.

The *Nursing Times* comment was: "It would appear that the training of the assistant nurse was being designed to meet the shortage of candidates rather than to prepare the candidate for the type of work which the assistant nurse ought to do, and in this connection the syllabus of examination also fills us with some misgiving"[13].

The Minister deferred approval of the syllabus of training until the Rules relating to the examination were also ready.

The names of the two Inspectors were announced in the summer of 1944. They were Miss B. Gebhard, S.R.N., formally Matron, Central Middlesex County Hospital, and Miss W. M. L. Selmes, S.R.N., D.N., Sister Tutor, Whiston County Hospital, Prescott, Lancs.

By the end of 1944, 9,556 applications for admission to the Roll had been received and by February 1945, 3,826 had been admitted with new names being added at about seven hundred to eight hundred a month.

At the Council meeting in January 1945, the names of the first hospitals to be approved provisionally as training schools for assistant nurses, were announced. They were all in Essex:

St. Margarets Hospital, Epping
St. Johns Hospital, Chelmsford
St. Andrews Hospital, Billericay
Orsett Lodge Hospital, Orsett, Grays.

TEACHERS OF NURSES

When nurse training had first been organised in 1860, Miss Nightingale had seen the need for some form of specific instruction; in her mind, the teaching function had been linked with the position of Home Sister who was responsible for the probationers' welfare and well-being. In some ways this was unfortunate since for years, theoretical instruction and the nurses home were indivisable, and the tutor found herself in the hospital hierarchy and responsible to the matron for many non-educational matters.

In 1914 Miss Gullan was appointed the first Sister-Tutor*, whose sole function was teaching, and from then on other hospitals, somewhat reluctantly, followed suit. During the late 1920s and early 1930s various colleges started courses for Sister Tutors, and awarded certificates to successful candidates. The first "specialised" section of the College of Nursing was the Sister Tutor Section, founded in 1925.

By the time the war started, it was realised that some form of

* At St. Thomas's Hospital.

registration for nurse teachers was desirable and in 1942 a letter was received from the Secretary of the Nurses Salaries Committee (Rushcliffe Committee) asking whether the Council would undertake to be the body responsible for the recognition of the Sister Tutors, and for regularising their status and conditions of training. The General Nursing Council were in favour of this, but pointed out that it would require new legislation; they did however, already recognise certain certificates:

The Royal College of Nursing Nurse-Teachers Certificate

King's College of Household and Social Science Certificate, Battersea Polytechnic Certificate

Certificate of Bedford College Course in combination with the Royal College of Nursing

Leeds University Sister Tutor Certificate, and the

Diploma of Nursing (teaching) of London or Leeds University.

Also in 1942, the Minister wrote to the Council to ask for their views on modifying the Act to provide the necessary powers. The Board of Education indicated that it was prepared to accept the holders of the above certificates as teachers of anatomy and physiology in pre-nursing courses.

Part 3 (14) of the 1943 Nurses Act laid down that "the power of the Council . . . shall extend to the making of Rules providing for the giving of certificates by or under the authority of the Council, to persons who have undergone the prescribed training (being training carried out in an institution approved by the Council in that behalf) and, if the Rules so provide, passed the prescribed examinations in the teaching of nursing"[14].

In July 1943, the Council set up an ad hoc committee to draft the Rules. By March 1944 an outline was approved by Council and it was decided to approach London University on the subject. Conferences were held during 1944, with interested bodies, and London University said that it was prepared, in principle, to set up a Diploma for Sister Tutors and to prescribe a scheme of training and examination. At the September Council meeting (1944) the rules were made public. Council were prepared to grant a certificate if:

(a) Application was made in writing.

(b) The candidate was on either the general register, or the part of the register for male nurses.

(c) The candidate had four years' post-registration experience (two as a sister in charge of a ward in an approved training school for student nurses).

(d) The candidate had completed a two years' Sister Tutor Course—provided that, until a date was announced by Council, a course of one year's duration be deemed sufficient.

(e) The candidate held a Sister Tutor Certificate issued by a University approved by Council.

(f) The candidate paid a fee of 3 guineas when the Council's certificate was granted.

When the Council's certificate was granted, a distinguishing mark would be placed against the candidates entry in the Register.

REGISTRATION AND THE LIST

The work of the Registration Department was made considerably more difficult at the outbreak of war, due to the movement of nurses. In September 1940, the Council approved 39 applications for new badges, from nurses who had lost the originals at or near Dunkirk, and 21 applications from those who had lost badges during the evacuation of the British Expeditionary Force from France.

In November 1940 Council decided to retain, without fee, the names of 165 nurses on the Register, since they were in enemy-occupied territory and unable to pay the annual retention fee. Throughout 1941, many similar requests for duplicate badges and certificates, lost as a result of enemy action, were received and granted.

The list

In 1933, Mr. Batey, M.P., introduced a Bill in the House of Commons to amend the Registration Act with regard to existing nurses. He said that 20,000 nurses had failed to register during the period of grace, and that the Registers should be opened again for one year to admit, without examination, properly trained nurses. The Bill was financed by the Mental Hospitals and Institutional Workers' Union, and at the time was opposed by the majority of registered nurses; it had a second reading on April 12th, at which it was blocked, and was subsequently deferred five times[15]. Although nothing came of this Bill the subject remained in the background and occasional letters appeared in the press. In the Nurses Act 1943 (18) there was provision for a list of "certain nurses not registered or enrolled". The nurses "are any persons, who within two years from the passing of this Act, apply for admission to the list, who hold certificates issued by institutions which appear to the Council to be satisfactory for the purposes of this provision, stating that they completed, before the beginning of July 1925, a course of training in nursing in the institution and who satisfy the Council that they are of good character and have adequate knowledge and experience of nursing"[16].

When the list was opened the Council set up a sub-committee to deal with applications. It was agreed that the requirements for admission to the list should be:

(a) Every applicant had to produce a certificate of training.

(b) The minimum would be a certificate of one year's training followed by two years bona fide nursing before November 1st, 1919. Certain exceptions would include those trained at St. Thomas's Hospital to whom no certificates were issued.

(c) There would be no admission to the list by virtue of experience only.

(d) The list would be open to nurses who were eligible to register during the periods of grace.

By 1945, over 4,000 enquiries had been received, and by November of that year some 2,200 applications had been approved and names added to the list. In the immediate post war years, applications were considered from nurses who had been in occupied countries, especially Jersey and Guernsey, at the time the list was opened. A scrutiny of the applications is fascinating: many were from men, and the majority of applicants trained between 1910 and 1920. Some were considerably earlier than this—dated 1899, 1900, 1901, 1902, 1904, and 1905. The list formed an appendix to the Register; it closed on April 22nd, 1945.

DISCIPLINE

In the early part of the war, the Council became concerned at the practice of registered nurses allowing their names to be used in the advertising of commercial products. In 1941 it was decided that this was to be classified as misconduct which could result in the nurse's name being removed from the Register. An announcement was made to this effect, and laid down what was permitted: Council approved advertising "by door plate, showing name, professional qualifications and address. By use of professional cards and stationery giving name, professional qualifications, address and telephone number. By advertisements in the press, including medical and nursing journals; such advertisements to be limited to name, professional qualifications, address, telephone number and nature of work desired. By calling upon or writing to registered medical practitioners, hospitals, nursing homes, nursing co-operations and other nursing institutions". This came into force on May 1st, 1941.

During the war the work of the Disciplinary and Penal Cases Committee increased slowly. Seventy-nine cases were considered, 31 names removed from the Register and seven names restored.

THE OFFICE AND STAFF

As with all other organisations, the work of the office during the war was made increasingly difficult by shortage of staff. Fortunately 23 Portland Place suffered little actual damage during the air raids: in September 1940, a nearby time-bomb necessitated evacuation of the premises for two days and at the subsequent Council meeting Dr. Evans was thanked for the loan of rooms in his home, as temporary accommodation. In May 1941 many windows were broken by blast and at the next meeting £100 was set aside for "future replacement of windows of the offices". In October 1941 it was decided to begin Council meetings at 2 p.m. instead of 2.30 p.m. because of the blackout; in the same month, Marylebone Council gave up the use of that part of the basement which had previously been requisitioned as air-raid shelters.

In May 1942 Council considered the form of the minutes of all its meetings, and approved "that the Minutes of Council retain their present form and constitute a record of work done; that all resolutions or amendments proposed and seconded be included, but that detailed discussion in committee be not

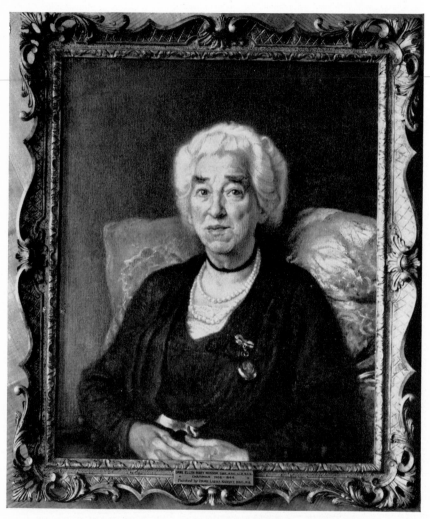

13. Dame Ellen Musson (from the portrait in the Council Chamber).

recorded in the minutes". This last is obviously a wise precaution but is frustrating to researchers!

During 1943 Council applied to the Ministry to increase the senior staff by the addition of a second assistant registrar. The Ministry took this opportunity for its officials to discuss the staffing of the office and methods of work. The new appointment was approved, and Miss M. Henry, S.R.N., was appointed. When Dame Ellen visited the Ministry she was told that the report on the work of the office was highly complimentary. The Council members congratulated the staff on this satisfactory state of affairs. In the same year the General Purposes Committee reported that a revision of the scale of staff salaries, which had been in operation since 1926, had been carried out and a new and greatly improved scale of salaries introduced.

PERSONALITIES

Until the end of 1943, Dame Ellen continued as Chairman of Council and Miss D. M. Smith was Vice-Chairman. In January 1943, Dame Ellen "confessed she had been disappointed that her term of office had not ended automatically with a departure from the Council in 1940; but she realised that the other members were very busy and that this was a way in which she could help. If they would put up with age and infirmity—which were both increasing—she would continue". However in January 1944 she retired from being Chairman and her place was taken by Miss D. M. Smith. Her resignation was received with deep regret and the comment was made: "The General Nursing Council meeting this week was a historic occasion. It saw the termination of a unique contribution to the development of the nursing profession"[17]. Dame Ellen Musson, D.B.E., R.R.C., LL.D., was one of the early nurses to apply for State Registration and was S.R.N. No. 26. She became a member of Council at the first election in 1923, and the first nurse Chairman of Council in 1926. She continued in this office until the end of 1943 and was Vice-Chairman in 1944. At the January 1944 Council meeting a resolution was passed: "that this Council places on record its deep appreciation of and gratitude for Dame Ellen Musson's outstanding work, not only for the General Nursing Council but also for the nursing profession as a whole. Most especially the Council would stress its appreciation of her wise and vigorous chairmanship throughout the past 18 years, of the high standard which she has always set and of the way in which she has given so generously of her time and talents. Dame Ellen is resigning the Chairmanship, but the work of future Councils will be built securely on the strong foundations she has laid during her years of office". The following members paid individual tribute: Miss Dey, Miss MacManus, Dr. Macaulay, Dr. Rees Thomas, Mr. Buckley and Miss Pearce, and a letter was read from Miss Cox-Davies who unfortunately was ill. Dame Ellen expressed her thanks and replied, "it was more years than she cared to count since she sat as a probationer in the old library at St. Bartholomew's and resolved to do all that was possible for the nurse in training. It had been a long struggle beginning with the first step with Mrs. Fenwick, Miss Isla Stewart and others to get the Registration of Nurses in 1919 and the economic reform which had since taken place".

After the Council meeting a tea party was held and Dame Ellen was presented with a fur cape.

During the war the announcement of the deaths of many early Council members were made. Dr. E. W. Goodall (1938), Miss M. E. Sparshott (1940), and Sir Joseph Priestley, the first Chairman (1941). Dame Alicia Lloyd Still, D.B.E., R.R.C., S.R.N. (No. 2) died in September 1944; she had trained at St. Thomas's Hospital in 1895, became Matron of the Brompton Hospital in 1904, Matron of the Middlesex Hospital in 1909, and was Matron of St. Thomas's from 1913 till her retirement in December 1937; she was an appointed member of the first (Caretaker) Council and an elected member until 1937; she was Chairman of the Education and Examinations Committee from its inception until her retirement. In October 1944 Miss A. M. Bushby died. She was the elected representative of Sick Children's nurses at the first election in 1923 and remained on the Council until 1932. She was a staunch member of the British College of Nurses and an ardent supporter of Mrs. Fenwick.

Also in October 1944 the death was announced of Miss R. A. Cox-Davies, C.B.E., R.R.C. and bar, S.R.N. (No. 3). Miss Cox-Davies trained at St. Bartholomew's Hospital 1893-6 and was a sister in her training school; in 1903 she became Matron of the Royal Devon and Exeter Hospital, and of the Royal Free Hospital, London, in 1905; she retired from hospital work in

1922; she was an appointed member of the first (Caretaker) Council and an elected member until the time of her death; she was Vice-Chairman of Council 1928–31, 1933–4, and 1938.

The first Registrar, Miss M. S. Riddell died in St. Bartholomew's Hospital in September 1941. When this was announced at the Council meeting Dame Ellen said: "it would be difficult to estimate the value of her work to the whole nursing profession and to the public whom they serve".

An unusual tribute was paid at the end of 1939 when the death of Miss Margaret Breay was announced at a Council meeting. Miss Breay (S.R.N. No. 13) was a lifelong friend and supporter of Mrs. Fenwick and indeed her name appears as a referee on Mrs. Fenwick's application for registration. Miss Breay trained at St. Bartholomew's Hospital and subsequently made her career in nursing journalism, and joined the staff of the *British Journal of Nursing*. She reported all Council meetings for this journal, until her death, and Dame Ellen paid tribute to the accuracy of her reporting, and said that future historians would be grateful to her. It is quite true that for the first 20 years of its existence the fullest records of the Council's meetings are to be found in the *British Journal of Nursing*.

In 1942, members' term of office came to an end officially, and although no election was held the new appointed members were announced. They were:

Ministry of Health: Dr. W. Russell Brain, D.M., F.R.C.P. (The London Hospital).

Dr. H. M. C. Macaulay, B.Sc., M.D., D.P.H. (County Medical Officer of Health, L.C.C.).

Professor Ralph M. S. Picken, M.B., Ch.B., D.P.H.

Dr. W. Rees Thomas, M.D., F.R.C.P., D.P.M.

Miss K. C. Watt, C.B.E., R.R.C., S.R.N. (First Chief Nursing Officer, Ministry of Health).

Privy Council: Countess of Limerick, Sir Henry Gooch, both re-appointed.

Board of Education: Mr. H. M. Walton, M.A. (Secretary, Middlesex Local Education Authority).

Miss A. Catnach, B.A. (Headmistress, Putney County Secondary School).

THE ELECTION

In October 1941, an application was made to the Privy Council "that steps be taken to extend the term of office of the present Council by a period of one year". It was felt that it was not desirable to attempt to hold an election in the middle of the war. In May 1942 the Minister of Health sent a copy of the Order in Council, extending the term of office of the elected members by one year. At a later date this was extended further and the election finally took place at the end of 1944.

The notices of election were sent to the national and nursing press in July 1944, and the addresses in the books of the Council on July 31st, 1944 were used for the electorate; the ballot papers were sent out "on or about October 31st, 1944". The press exhorted nurses to use their votes and it was noted that Dame Ellen was not standing for re-election—she was now 77 years old.

Thirty-seven candidates stood for the 16 seats:

24 for the eleven general seats.

3 ,, ,, one male nurses seat.

3 ,, ,, one female mental nurses seat.

3 ,, ,, one male mental nurses seat.

2 ,, ,, one sick children's nurses seat.

2 ,, ,, one fever nurses seat.

This was the first time there had been more than one candidate for the fever nurses representative and the last election at which this group had direct representation.

All those members of Council who stood for re-election were elected and there were five new members. The results were as follows:

General seats: *votes*

Miss E. Pearce,   17,713   re-elected

Miss E. E. P. Mac-
    Manus   16,312   re-elected.

Miss C. H. Alexander	16,086	Matron, The London Hospital, London
Miss H. Dey,	15,120	re-elected
Miss M. Jones	14,482	re-elected
Miss D. M. Smith	14,288	re-elected
Miss G. V. L. Hillyers	14,174	Matron, St. Thomas's Hospital, London
Miss L. G. D. Grant	13,819	re-elected.
Miss M. Houghton	13,703	Principal Tutor, University College Hospital, London
Miss D. L. Holland	13,327	Tutor, Guy's Hospital, London
Miss J. M. Calder	13,070	Chief Nursing Officer, London County Council

Male nurse:
Mr. F. A. W. Craddock   190

Mental nurse:

Mr. J. H. Buckley	1,196	re-elected
Miss K. M. Willis	1,170	re-elected

Sick Children's nurse:
Miss D. A. Lane   1,464   re-elected

Fever nurses:
Miss F. M. Campbell   1,960   re-elected

Of those eleven elected as representing the general part of the Register, ten were from teaching hospitals—eight in London. The returning officer reported that as well as the valid nominations, one had been received with no form of declaration of consent and efforts to rectify this were not successful. The total electorate was 119,586 and the Post Office were unable to deliver 1,653 letters; there were 2,495 invalid votes and 803 voting papers were returned too late. The total number of valid votes cast was 43,737—37 per cent of the electorate who received voting papers.

The new members of Council took office in January 1945.

References

1. *Nursing Times*—29.13.38.
2. Ibid—4.5.40.

3. Ibid—2.11.40.
4. Ibid—7.10.36.
5. Ibid—18.2.37.
6. Nursing Reconstruction Committee—(Horder).
7. Nurses Act 1943.
8. Ibid.
9. Ibid.
10. *Nursing Times*—17.4.43.
11. Select Committee on the Registration of Nurses 1905.
12. *Nursing Times*—19.2.44.
13. Ibid—8.7.44.
14. Nurses Act 1943.
15. *British Journal of Nursing*—3.4.33.
16. Nurses Act 1943.
17. *Nursing Times*—5.2.44.

Chapter 8

THE POST-WAR YEARS, 1945–1950

"There is, however, no advantage in reflections on the past further than may be of service to the present". THUCYDIDES

EDUCATION AND EXAMINATIONS

Examinations

At the beginning of 1945, the Council decided to revert to the pre-war practice of holding the examinations three times a year, in February, June and October. The number of candidates was some 26,000 a year which made the Council one of the largest examining bodies in the country. As from February 1946 all candidates for admission to the Final Examination had to have completed the prescribed training by the last day of the month in which the written examination was held, and attained the age of 21 years—in the case of the Fever Final Examination, 20 years. In 1946, various sub-committees were set up to consider the examinations, and comprehensive training; a regulation was made that any candidate who failed the Final Examination three times, must undertake six months further training.

From June 1950, changes were made in both the Preliminary and Final Examinations; for both examinations, the orals (in anatomy, physiology, hygiene and medicine and surgery) were discontinued, but the time allowed for the practical part of the examinations was increased—the Preliminary from 30 to 40 minutes and the Final from 40 minutes to one hour.

When the Royal Medico-Psychological Association handed over responsibility for their examinations of mental nurses to the Council, they insisted on the inclusion of Psychology in the Part 2, Preliminary Examination syllabus. The Minister agreed to this and the subject was an optional one from June 1950 and compulsory from October 1951.

War-time auxiliaries

Much discussion went on over the position of those men and women who had undertaken nursing work in the armed forces, the Civil Nursing Reserve, the British Red Cross Society and the St. John Ambulance Brigade, and their subsequent position

149

with regard to further training. Those auxiliaries who had had not less than two years experience of nursing the sick in hospital under the supervision of trained nurses could, if recommended by the Matron of the hospital, receive six months reduction in training for the Register. This concession was retrospective to the outbreak of war but candidates had to apply within six months of discharge from the services mentioned.

The Ministry of Health, with the approval of Council, set up one year, intensive courses, which led to the examination for State Registration, for those who had held specified nursing ranks in the forces. Both these concessions continued until October 31st, 1953.

Nurse-training

It had long been realised that the Council had no accurate records as to the numbers entering and leaving nurse training, since no official forms were required until a student entered for the Preliminary Examination. It had been assumed that wastage was high, but no national statistics were available. At the end of the war it was decided that index forms should be required from February 1946 for pupil nurses, and from June 1947 for student nurses at the beginning of training, and discontinuation forms when nurses left without completing training. From June 1947—May 1950, 59,722 students entered training and 17,596 withdrew, of whom 3,025 re-entered: (see appendix 5(iii)). It was noted that wastage was highest in the psychiatric hospitals and higher amongst male students than among female students.

The war had either stopped or held up a number of improvements that the Council wished to implement, and the new Council set about attempting to get Ministerial approval on several points. They must have felt singularly frustrated when, in November 1945, a letter was received from the Minister, containing the following: The Minister was unable to agree to a post registration part of the register for tuberculosis nurses, or for orthopaedic nurses; he felt the time was not opportune for an increase in the minimum age of entry for nurse training; he felt the re-introduction of a test examination would seriously affect recruitment; he wanted more information about the work involved in the registration of tutors; he did not feel prepared to agree to an increase in the fees for certificates; he pointed out that not all hospitals could have Preliminary Training Schools by May 1947, due to the building restrictions, and, therefore, the Council should inform hospital authorities that the time limit would be extended; and he was apprehensive that the Council's new proposals for the approval of training schools (daily average of 100 occupied beds from June 1947) would aggravate the shortage of nurses, and suggested each training school should be considered on its merits[1].

It is at such times that detailed records of discussion in committee would be invaluable but it is stated that Council agreed to discuss the letter with the Minister.

One of the controversial matters came to a head during 1947 and 1948. In August 1947, questions were asked in the House of Commons about the number of hospitals from which the Council had withdrawn approval as training schools during the past year. The answer was, 23 voluntary and one municipal hospital. Asked how many further hospitals would lose approval shortly, the reply was 25 voluntary and 12 municipal. M.P.'s were concerned about the position of the smaller and specialised hospitals—especially fever hospitals—and the Minister, Mr. Aneurin Bevan, said he would keep the matter in mind.

In January 1948 the Council decided "that in so far as hospitals approved as training schools for fever nurses are concerned, the Council's requirement regarding the daily average occupation of beds be not implemented at the present time".

One hospital appealed, under the Act, against withdrawal of approval; this was St. Leonards Hospital, Shoreditch, London. The appeal was heard by Mr. V. Zachary Cope, F.R.C.S., and Miss M. F. Dykes, S.R.N., R.F.N., S.C.M. The Minister allowed the appeal and overruled the Council. He said that, judging by the results of the General Nursing Council's examinations over a period of years (73 per cent of passes—three nurses being successful at a recent examination), the nurse-training had been efficient. He thought that complaints about accommodation, amenities, sanitary arrangements and repair of buildings were justified and the Council could urge improvements. The conditions had not, he contended, had a serious effect on the health or training of the nurses but might have slightly increased the wastage; this was given as 49 per cent. The

Minister suggested a long list of necessary improvements at the hospital and said he would give assistance. While the improvements were being carried out he "allowed that the hospital continue to be an approved training school". In April 1948, the Council set up an ad hoc committee to consider the procedure in cases which involved withdrawal of approval of a training school.

By June 1947 all training schools were expected to have introduced Preliminary Training Schools of at least eight weeks in length. For those psychiatric hospitals which had difficulty in implementing this, the time limit was extended.

A sub-committee was set up to revise the syllabuses of subjects for examination which had remained unchanged since 1932.

The Education and Examinations Committee felt that the future of affiliated schemes and fever training were in some doubt and much discussion took place on these points.

Inspectors of training schools

In December 1944 the Council announced with regret that it was no longer possible for its members to carry out inspections of training schools every five years. In April 1945 they approached the Minister for approval of two posts of salaried inspectors for training schools for student nurses. They wished the matter reviewed in six months time with a possibility of increasing the number of posts, and recommended a starting salary of £425 a year. The Ministry approved this on a temporary basis.

The first two inspectors to be appointed were Miss M. E. Craven, R.R.C., S.R.N., who trained at the General Infirmary at Leeds from 1917–22 and was Matron of The Peace Memorial Hospital at Watford, Herts, and Miss M. G. Gill, S.R.N., who trained at University College Hospital from 1916–19, and had just retired from being Matron of Hornsey Central Hospital since 1931.

By 1950 the inspectorate had risen to five and an Education Officer had been appointed. The Council's Inspectors were required to wear State Registered uniform when on duty.

TEACHERS OF NURSES

In April 1945 the Council approved the whole-time one-year course for tutors at the University of London, for the session

1945-46. They agreed that those obtaining the Diploma should be entitled to receive the Council's certificate of registration as a Sister-Tutor.

They later gave similar approval to the Universities of Birmingham, Manchester, Hull and Leeds.

By October 1947, 313 tutors had applied for registration. In October 1949 Council agreed that from October 1950, the course at London University would be of two years' duration.

MENTAL NURSES

In May 1939 the Council received a letter from Sir Arthur Hall, Chairman of the mental sub-committee of the Inter-departmental (Athlone) Committee on nursing services.

He asked if the Council would reconsider the situation with regard to mental nurses' registration. The sub-committee felt that there was a conflict between the examination systems of the Council and the R.M.P.A. If agreement could not be reached, it was felt that perhaps a separate statutory body should be established to register all mental nurses. The Council appointed its own mental committee to consider the matter. The following month, a letter was read from the secretary of the Society of Registered Male Nurses, regretting the Athlone Committee's suggestions and saying they would do all in their power to oppose them. They suggested that all the supplementary registers should be swept away and there should be one register of nurses. Dame Ellen said there was sometimes a misapprehension about the Register—it was one Register, the Register of Nurses, although it had six parts.

The Mental Nurses Committee continued to meet and in 1944, reported the formation of a sub-committee to discuss a revision of the examination syllabus for registered mental nurses and registered nurses of mental defectives.

In 1945, representatives of the Council and the R.M.P.A. met, and correspondence and discussion were resumed. In January 1946 the report of the Athlone sub-committee on mental nursing was published. It recommended:

(1) That there should in future be one accepted qualifying examination for the mental nurse. It noted that between 1936 and 1938, 5,600 nurses entered for the R.M.P.A. examination and 613 for the Council's examination—and wondered why.

The committee felt that mental hospital authorities and medical superintendents were conservative and had not encouraged nurses to take the State examinations. State Registration brought no financial reward, and the Council's examination was more difficult and more expensive than that of the R.M.P.A.

(2) That there should be more representation by mental nurses on the Council. The present mental nurses committee could not have a majority of mental nurses and although mental nurses on the Council agreed that their opinion had always prevailed, this might not happen in future. There should be five mental nurses on the Council, three elected and two appointed.

Discussions continued between the Council, the R.M.P.A., and the Board of Control. In August 1946 the R.M.P.A. issued a statement:

"The most important announcement to the mental nursing profession; the cessation of their examinations. In agreement with the General Nursing Council for England and Wales, candidates will not be accepted for training after December 31st, 1946. Those holding the R.M.P.A. final certificates will be entered on the appropriate parts of the State Register on application to the General Nursing Council before December 31st, 1951. The General Nursing Council agree to approve those schools of nursing approved by the Association"[2].

The nursing press welcomed this development and said that all would acknowledge the debt that the mental nursing world owed to the R.M.P.A. The announcement followed the recommendations of both the Athlone Committee and the Horder Reconstruction Committee.

At the end of 1946 the Council delegated power to the Mental Nurses Committee to approve hospitals as training schools for mental and mental defective nurses, but not power to withdraw approval.

It was agreed that holders of the R.M.P.A. certificate need not take the Preliminary State Examination, if undergoing training for another part of the Register.

After some consultation between the Council and the Ministry, it was agreed that the final date for applications from holders of the R.M.P.A. certificate to be placed on the Register should be extended to March 31st, 1952.

In January 1948 the Minister approved the Rules relating to the admission to the Register for Mental nurses; he agreed that, pending legislation for a mental nurses' Board, five persons with mental qualifications should be appointed by him as "assessors" to attend meetings of the mental nurses committee, to express views and offer advice.

The notices reminding mental nurses to register were sent to the press by the Council in January 1948. After further discussion the closing date for applications was waived. The last examination was conducted by the R.M.P.A. in November 1951 and the new Nurses Rules came into effect in August 1951. The fee charged for initial registration was two guineas, except for those nurses whose names appeared on the List, who were to pay one guinea. The entry on the Register was marked "by virtue of M.P.A.", if the certificate was issued before 1925, and "by virtue of R.M.P.A." if issued after that date.

In over 80 years the Royal Medico-Psychological Association had issued some 48,000 certificates in mental nursing and some 4,700 in mental deficiency nursing. An eminent doctor who was involved in much of the negotiations said in 1961: "Looking back, it seems to me that much of what we (the R.M.P.A.) did in a fruitless effort to defeat the General Nursing Council's policy was misguided and a little childish. On the other hand, I think we did well to maintain our own examination in being, until after the last war, for in this way we eventually secured entry to the Register for a large number of nurses who would otherwise have remained unrecognised. . . . We clung to our own system, not because it was the best, but because it seemed to offer a better chance of reform"[3].

The 1949 Nurses Act made provision for the establishment of a Mental Nurses Committee, to consider:

(a) Any matter which wholly or mainly concerns registered mental nurses (other than disciplinary matters).

(b) Any matter relating to the training of persons (for the mental registers).

The Committee were to report on the above matters to Council, who having considered the report, could take action. As with the Assistant Nurses Committee, the Council were empowered to delegate authority on a particular matter, if they so wished[4]. One difference between the statutory powers of this and the Assistant Nurses Committee, is that the latter were given power in 1943 to deal with disciplinary matters.

The composition of the Mental Nurses Committee was laid down in the third schedule to the 1949 Act. It was to consist of 12 persons:

(a) Six members of Council, appointed by the Council, of whom two were to be the elected mental nurses.

(b) Two were to be registered mental nurses elected to the Committee by registered mental nurses.

(c) Four were to be appointed by the Minister.

One, a matron of a mental hospital which was an approved training school.

One, a registered mental nurse, engaged in teaching in an approved training school.

One, a registered medical practitioner engaged in the teaching of psychiatry, and

One, a chief male nurse of a hospital which was an approved training school.

The term of office of the Committee was to be five years[5].

ASSISTANT NURSES

In 1945, a uniform sub-committee was set up to consider the question of the official uniform for State Enrolled Assistant Nurse (S.E.A.N.).

At the end of the year, reminders were published in the press, that existing assistant nurses had only until February 3rd, 1946 to enrol. The first election of the Assistant Nurses Committee was due to be held in May 1946, but in view of "the delay in admitting nurses to the Roll" the Committee suggested that the Minister should be asked to postpone the election for three years to enable more nurses to vote. Council agreed, but the Minister felt it better to have an extension to May 31st, 1947 and a further extension later, if necessary. By the end of 1946 there were 24,612 nurses on the Roll.

The rules for training for enrolment were published in 1946. The training was to be for two years and was to be of a practical nature. There was to be a four-week Preliminary Training School. The first year was to be spent in a hospital for the chronic sick and all women pupils were to have experience nursing men, women, and children. In the second year it was suggested that the pupils could spend nine months in a special hospital such as a sanatorium or fever hospital.

The examination was to be three times a year—in March, July and November. The theoretical part of the examination was to be on the lines of the quiz system—that is, the type of question where a sentence had to be completed. The practical part was to be held in the wards and candidates had to have worked, in the ward where they were to be assessed, for at least one month before the examination. There were to be two assessors for four to six candidates, and the time for the practical was not to exceed one and a half hours.

Recruitment of pupil nurses was disappointingly slow in the early days and in April 1946 only about one hundred were indexed.

There was much controversy in the profession over the content of the pupil nurses' practical training. Some felt it was too broad and included procedures which ought to be the province of the S.R.N.—e.g. the administration of oxygen.

The Committee suggested a reduction of six months' training for certain intermediate and existing assistant nurses who had nursing experience during the war; this was approved.

Council agreed with the Minister that the Roll of Assistant Nurses (intermediate) should remain open for one year longer than planned, until January 1st, 1949. The Committee were reluctant to agree, but felt that they must, in view of the small number of training schools for pupil nurses which had been established; the extension of the date meant that hospitals were able to recruit unqualified nurses, who on completion of the necessary two years' training or experience, would be eligible to enrol as assistant nurses (intermediate).

In 1947, the Council re-opened the Roll for existing assistant nurses, since many who had failed to enrol were finding difficulty in obtaining work, due to the restriction on the title nurse and assistant nurse in the 1943 Act.

By May 1947, 72 training schools for pupil nurses had been approved and by November 1949, 128 (see appendix 5(v)).

The election for the Assistant Nurses Committee was finally held in 1948. Notices were sent to the press. Nineteen valid nominations were received; one nomination was invalid since the nominator was not a State Enrolled Assistant Nurse. Ten of the nominees were men, but the four finally elected were women. The electorate was 37,511.

Those elected were:

Miss M. G. Burns, S.R.N.

Miss L. C. Avery, S.E.N.

Mrs. L. E. Charteris, S.E.N.

Mrs. V. N. E. Moss, S.R.N.

During 1948 the whole subject of training for the Roll was discussed and at one point serious consideration was given to its closure (see page 163).

However, it was decided to modify conditions of training and two major changes were made in the Rules. In October 1949, the Minister agreed that the requirement that one year should be spent nursing the chronic sick, should be dispensed with; any type of hospital could now apply for approval provided the conditions of training and teaching were satisfactory. The syllabus of subjects for examination was revised and could now be completed in one year; after the Test, the pupil had to work for a further year under supervision, before being enrolled. This change took place as from June 1st, 1950.

The first examination—called the Test for admission to the Roll—was held in 1949: 61 entered, two were absent and 59 were tested and passed. Six of this number were already S.E.A.N. and chose to take the Test for their own satisfaction. There were 17 centres.

A Ministry circular R.H.B. (49) 156, to hospital authorities, pointed out that there were now 1,400 pupil nurses in training, but 17,000 "other nursing staff". Hospitals were encouraged to establish pupil nurse training schools, since it was felt many of those in "other" grades would make excellent assistant nurses.

REGISTRATION

Early in 1945 it was suggested that instead of printing a full edition of the Register for that year, a schedule of additions and deletions to the Register for 1944 should be published; this was made necessary by shortage of staff, paper, and the delay caused by the refusal of the paper control to allow paper for the election.

In the 1943 Act, there was provision for the Minister to make regulations about the restriction of the title nurse and an order was made by him under Section 6 (1) Proviso (b) of the Nurses Act 1943; in 1945 this allowed certain groups of people to call themselves "trained nurse", "maternity nurse", "orthopaedic nurse", "children's nurse", etc., in specific circumstances. The first order, 2 (m) allowed "a person recognised by the body known as the Church of Christ Scientist, as being a member of that body and as qualified for employment by members of that body, as a Christian Science nurse (may) use the name or title of "Christian Science nurse". This lead to questions in the House of Commons and uproar in the profession. The Council were firm that the term nurse should not be used, and in April 1946 that part of the 1943 Act was annulled. In December 1946 the Chairman announced to Council that on November 29th a motion to permit the use of the title "Christian Science nurse" had been defeated in both Houses.

In 1947, the Minister made an Order under Section 6 (1) Proviso (b) for those nurses who qualified before July 1925, who through internment or other circumstances outside their control were not able to apply for inclusion in the List, to do so.

In the same year the Council were distressed to learn that the Registered Nurses' Association of British Columbia, Canada, "wish to terminate the agreement (reciprocal registration) on the grounds that the educational standard of entry to the profession, in Great Britain, was inadequate, and the standard of professional training not acceptable". It will be remembered that the Test Examination had been discontinued at the outbreak of the war and despite the Council's efforts had not yet been re-introduced. The Council notified the Minister of this development, and the Minister replied that he had learnt with regret the decision of the Association and he fully appreciated the importance of keeping up the standards of nurse training.

In 1948 the Minister was again approached about publishing a supplement to the Register each year. The 1947 Register had contained 130,000 names, was published in three volumes and cost £7,602; Council estimated an annual saving of £6,000 if this was allowed. The Minister agreed to include this change in the next Act. At the end of the same year, the Council had a conference of bodies representing nurses to discuss the cost of registration and a proposed change in the financial organisation of the Council. The proposals were:

(1) That a life retention fee of 3 guineas should be paid, with a smaller sum on a graded scale for existing members.

(2) That the examination fees should be raised.

It was pointed out that the annual retention fee was 2s. 6d. and it cost 4s. 5½d. to collect it in each case; also the number of nurses failing to pay each year was rising (over 5,000 a year).

In 1949 it was decided to issue the uniform permit and badge on receipt of the initial registration fee.

These changes, too, were incorporated in the 1944 Act and the Rules came into operation on March 24th, 1950.

FINANCE

Many of the Council's financial problems have just been outlined.

In 1944, part of the balance sheet read as follows:

	£	s.	d.
Expenditure	72,207	11	4
Excess of income over expenditure	2,560	13	1
Examination fees received	54,795	12	7
Examiners fees paid	33,643	14	7
(does not include costs of the examinations department).			

In 1946 it was announced that there was a balance of £1,163 9s. 4d., due to the fact that the 1945 Register had not been published.

By 1948 it was announced that in the previous financial year there was a deficit of £18,354 17s. 8d., and it was estimated that the deficit for the current year would be £33,000.

As previously mentioned a conference was held. Nineteen professional associations and unions with nurse members sent representatives. Miss Smith, Chairman of Council, said that proposals had been submitted to the Minister to remedy the situation. He was prepared to approve these if the profession agreed.

The proposed changes in the examination fees were:

Preliminary—£1 15s. instead of £1 10s. for each part.

Both parts £2 12s. 6d. instead of £2 2s.

Final—£4 4s. instead of £3 3s.

This was the first increase since 1939 and would cover the cost of the examinations and the maintenance of the Index.

The Minister had indicated that he was prepared to reimburse the Council for the cost of Inspection of training schools, but wanted comments by the end of 1948. This was one reason for holding the conference on December 14th. The cost of inspections at the time was £10,000 per year. Most of the delegates agreed with the proposals.

DISCIPLINE

During the period discussed (1945–50) disciplinary action was taken against 34 registered nurses and their names removed from the Register; judgement was postponed in 26 cases, and 13 were dismissed. Sixteen applications for the restoration of a name to the Register were granted.

The Assistant Nurses Committee took action against 14 nurses whose names were removed from the Roll and three cases were postponed; 13 persons were prosecuted for falsely claiming to be S.E.A.N.'s.

UNIFORM

The uniform committee carried out the first revision of the State Registered uniform since 1931 and designs submitted by Norman Hartnell were used.

THE WOOD REPORT

The social changes and legislation which took place in the mid-1940s made it essential for an appraisal of all services—including nursing. In January 1946, the Ministry of Health, the Department of Health for Scotland and the Ministry of Labour and National Service set up a working Party on the Recruitment and Training of Nurses. The members of the working party were: Sir Robert Wood, K.B.E., C.B., the Chairman; Miss D. C. Bridges, R.R.C., S.R.N., S.C.M.; Miss E. Cockayne, S.R.N., S.C.M.; Dr. J. Cohen, M.A., Ph.D., F.B.Ps.S.; and D. T. Inch, C.B.E., M.C., M.D., F.R.C.P. (Edin.), D.P.H. They were assisted by a steering committee, and secretaries and assistant secretaries. Their detailed report was published in 1947, and contained 40 main conclusions. Dr. Cohen published a minority report.

Those conclusions directly affecting the statutory body and nurse training were:

(1) The key problem in the present system is wastage during training (para. 88).

(2) Nurses in training must no longer be regarded as junior employees, but must be accorded full student status (para. 108).

(3) If student nurses were relieved of non-nursing duties and those duties dictated solely by the staffing demands of the hospitals, a period of two years would suffice for general training (paras. 122, 127).

(4) The two-year training would be based on a five-day, 40-hour week, with six weeks' annual holiday (para. 122).

(5) The first 18 months of training would be in the fundamentals common to all fields of nursing and the last six months in a chosen speciality (paras. 128–9, 133).

(6) Training must include social and preventive medicine (paras. 130, 136).

(7) The State Examination should be in two parts, one at the end of the first 18 months, on the content of the common course, and one at the end of two years, on the elective speciality (para. 139).

(8) The student who passed the second examination would register and receive the appropriate salary, but must complete a further year under supervision before being qualified to practise (para. 140).

(9) One common Register should replace the present general and supplementary parts of the Register (para. 144).

(10) If nurses in training were to have student status the following requirements must be met:
  (a) Adequate nursing and domestic staff.
  (b) The finance of nurse training should be independent of hospital finance.
  (c) Students should be under the control of the training authority and not of the hospital.
  (d) Recruitment should be the responsibility of the Health Departments (paras. 146–9).

(11) There must be adequate teaching staff, trained in modern educational methods (paras. 154–6).

(12) Regional Group training schools were recommended (para. 186).

(13) There should be Regional Nurse Training Boards whose duties would include the planning, and co-ordination of training facilities (paras. 193–6).

(14) There should be, within the Departments of Health, Nursing Advisory Committees to advise on nurse education and to have powers of inspection (paras. 197–8).

(15) Research units should be established within the Departments of Health (paras. 199–200).

(16) There should be one General Nursing Council for Great Britain. It should include governmental, university and other educational representatives, and nurses elected regionally (para. 204).

(17) The Roll of Assistant Nurses should be closed and their place taken by nursing orderlies (para. 250).

The Report had several appendices which contained a large amount of statistical evidence[6].

Dr. Cohen's minority report was published a year later. He wanted much more than a slow reform of present circumstances; his recommendations included:

(1) An even flow of suitable candidates, equally, to all training centres.

(2) Selection procedures to be devised and conducted by experts.

(3) The jurisdiction over State Examinations and teaching programmes should be given to the Health Departments.

(4) There should be a Committee of Inquiry into the future existence and role of the General Nursing Council.

Dr. Cohen conducted a small survey into some 100 S.R.N.s and compared their examination marks with their efficiency a year later, as judged by senior nursing staff. There were at this time some 125,000 Registered Nurses.

An *ad hoc* committee of the General Nursing Council considered the Report of the Wood Committee in great detail and published a memorandum of 11 foolscap sheets in 1948.

They agreed that wastage was a problem, but felt that the statistics given had been compiled in war time and were perhaps misleading. There was a great need for the re-introduction of an educational minimum standard of entry. They agreed that the age of entry should be 18 years.

They agreed that the nurse in training should have student status, and felt that a 48-hour week should include lectures, tutorial classes and time for private study.

They felt that 18 months' training and six months' special experience was quite inadequate. The working conditions suggested by the Wood Committee meant that the student nurse would work an equivalent of only 51, 30-hour weeks in hospital, during her two years' training.

They were sceptical about the possibility of effective supervision in the third year and felt the nurses' position might be abused.

They agreed in general with the suggested content of the training programme but felt that the time spent in each branch of nursing should be lengthened. The Council were of the opinion that provided the nurse in training was given the status of a student, was not required to do domestic work, and had a block or study day system, a comprehensive training could be undertaken in three years. If this could be established the supplementary parts of the Register could be closed, except for the Register for mental nurses.

They agreed that it was of paramount importance that the course of training must be dictated by the needs of the student nurse and not by the staffing requirements of the hospital.

They could not agree that the student should be under the control of a separate training authority.

They agreed with the need for adequate, well prepared teachers and were prepared to welcome experimental schemes of training. They felt the Council's powers should be widened to include experimentation and research.

On the reconstitution of the Council, they pointed out that the Minister of Health, the Privy Council and the Board of Education could appoint whom they wished.

They did not agree that the Roll should be closed, and felt that it was far too early to assess training for the Roll, which had only just started.

The memorandum ended, "in conclusion, the Council desires to draw the attention of the Minister to the fact that the report of the Working Party would appear to have been drawn up with insufficient thought of the needs of the patient which in fact form the basis on which any conclusions relating to nurse training must be built".

In ten years, three reports had been published (Athlone, Horder, and Wood) all attempting to solve the problems inherent in recruitment, selection, wastage, and training of nurses and the production of a stable trained staff.

The Council were only too aware of many of the defects and deficiencies but were in part hampered by the need for new legislation.

THE NURSES ACT 1949

The introduction of the National Health Service in 1948 was followed by the Nurses Act of 1949.

The Nurses Bill had its first reading in the House of Lords on April 12th, 1949 and reached the Committee stage by May 17th. It completed its passage in the Lords and was sent to the House of Commons as an agreed, non-party measure. The second reading in the Commons, and the Committee stage were in October and the Bill was welcomed by all speakers; the third and final reading was on November 4th and the day appointed for it to come into operation was January 1st, 1951. It was "an Act to reconstitute the General Nursing Council for England and Wales and otherwise to amend the Nurses Acts 1919–45, and to make further provision with respect to the training of nurses for the sick"[7]. It had four parts and four schedules.

Part 1 dealt with the reconstitution of the General Nursing Council.

Part 2 was concerned with nurse training and the setting up of Area Nurse-Training Committees and had six sections.

Part 3 was headed "miscellaneous amendments", and included details relating to a Finance Committee, a Mental Nurses Committee, registration of nurses trained abroad, approval of training schools, fees and allowances and other matters. It had 12 sections.

Part 4 contained supplementary provisions and had five sections.

The reconstitution of the Council

The new constitution was laid down in the first Schedule. There were to be 17 elected and 17 appointed members.

The 17 elected were to be as follows:

(a) Fourteen registered nurses (general or male nurses) elected by general or male nurses. One nurse was to be elected in each of 14 areas determined by the Minister. Fever nurses could vote in this section. Each of those nurses "shall, on the day of the election, be engaged, in the area for which he is elected, in nursing or in other work for which the employment of a registered nurse is requisite, or for which a registered nurse is commonly employed"[8].

(b) Two registered mental nurses, one male and one female, elected by registered mental nurses.

(c) One registered sick children's nurse, elected by registered sick children's nurses.

The 17 appointed were as follows:

(1) Twelve appointed by the Minister of Health.

    (a) Two registered nurses employed in "services provided under Part 3 of the National Health Service Act". (Local Authority Health Services.)

    (b) Two persons "holding certificates given by virtue of Section 14 of the Act of 1943" (Teachers of Nurses).

    (c) One male nurse.

    (d) One ward sister in an approved general training school.

    (e) Three persons "with experience in the control and management of hospitals".

This left three unspecified appointments.

(2) Three appointed by the Minister of Education.

(3) Two appointed by the Privy Council, one to represent Universities in England and Wales.

These changes increased the total membership of the Council from 25 to 34, and provided regional representation. The constitution insured that at least 23 seats were held by nurses.

Nurse training

(1) Committees were to be set up in each of the 14 areas, in consultation with the Council. The constitution of the Area Nurse-Training Committees was laid down in the second Schedule.

Each Committee was to consist of:

(*a*) Persons appointed by the Regional Hospital Board for the area.

(*b*) Persons appointed by Boards of Governors of teaching hospitals situated in the area.

(*c*) Persons appointed by the General Nursing Council.

(*d*) Persons appointed by the Central Midwives Board.

(*e*) Persons appointed by the Minister after consultation with the local health authorities in the area.

(*f*) Persons appointed by the Minister after consultation with such universities as he thinks fit.

(*g*) Persons appointed by the Minister after consultation with the local education authorities in the area.

The duties of the Area Nurse-Training Committees were laid down. They were to:

(*a*) Have regard to methods of nurse training within their area.

(*b*) Promote research and investigations into nurse training and to report the results to Council.

(*c*) Advise and assist Hospital Management Committees and Boards of Governors and others within the area, in the preparation and carrying out of schemes of training.

(*d*) Advise and assist the Council on matters relating to the approval of training schools in the area.

(*e*) Carry out other functions—e.g. examinations—if authorised to do so by the Council.

(2) The Council were given power to approve experimental schemes of training subject to the Minister's approval. These were to be any training schemes which differed from those laid down in the Acts of 1919 and 1943.

(3) Expenditure "wholly or mainly, for the purposes of or in connection with, the training of nurses" and as specified by the Minister, would be defrayed by Area Nurse Training Committees in accordance with approved estimates.

Miscellaneous amendments

(1) The Act stated that Council should appoint a Finance Committee, consisting of members of Council and two persons nominated by the Minister after consultation with the Council. All matters relating to Area Nurse-

Training Committee expenditure were to be referred to this committee, who would report back to the Council who would then take the necessary action.

(2) The Act stated that the Council should establish a Mental Nurses Committee (see page 155).

(3) The Council were given powers to register nurses trained abroad, or to suggest a period of further training and possibly examination before registration. This section also repealed sub-sections (1) and (2) of Section 6 of the 1919 Act which provided for the registration of nurses registered in any part of the Dominions.

(4) The male nurses' part of the Register was to be amalgamated with the general part of the Register.

(5) Power was given to the Council to request the Minister to close parts of the Register other than the general or male nurses part. This was so worded as to refer only to the fever part of the Register.

(6) Provisions relating to the approval of training institutions were changed. The Council, if considering withdrawal of approval, had to state its grounds in writing to the management of the institution. They also had to allow representatives of the management to put their views in writing and to appear before the Council to be heard, if they wished. Appeals against the Council's decisions were now to be made in writing to the Permanent Secretary to the Lord Chancellor who would set up the necessary machinery. This repealed subsection (2) of section 7 of the Act of 1919 and subsection (2) of section 5 of the Act of 1943, which provided the right of appeal to the Minister.

(7) The Act allowed the Council to charge those responsible for the management of hospitals not within the Health Service (disclaimed hospitals) for inspection and approval. The Minister could now contribute towards the cost of inspection and approval of National Health Service hospitals.

(8) The Council were to make rules providing for the admission to the Register of those persons whose names were on the list. The list was re-opened on the same basis as before.

(9) As already described, provision was made for the abolition of the annual retention fee and the change in the publication of the Register.

Several other minor matters were covered and in the supplementary provisions the Council were directed to make an annual report to the Minister as to the discharge by them of their functions with respect to the training of nurses, which should be laid before Parliament.

THE OFFICE AND STAFF

At the beginning of 1945 Council discussed an extension to the premises at 23 Portland Place and set up a Housing Committee. In May 1945, the Committee recommended that 17 Portland Place should be purchased; this was done and the flat and garage at 17 Duchess Mews, which were part of the property, were let.

The Registrar

During 1945, the Registrar, Miss G. E. Davies, became ill and although she returned to her post she obviously decided to retire, since in June 1946 it was announced that the Registrar's post would become vacant in May 1947, and advertisements were sent to the press. During Miss Davies' absence on sick leave Miss M. G. N. Henry, assistant Registrar, was authorised to act as Registrar to the Council. In December 1946 the following announcement appeared: "Miss M. G. N. Henry, S.R.N., S.C.M., first assistant Registrar to the General Nursing Council, has been appointed Registrar following the resignation of Miss G. E. Davies on account of ill-health. Miss Henry is a trainee of University College Hospital, London, W.C.1 and was appointed second assistant Registrar in April 1943 and first assistant Registrar in August 1944. Miss Henry will take up her duties on January 1st, 1947. We congratulate her upon her appointment. At the meeting of the General Nursing Council on November 29th (1946), the members recorded their very deep appreciation of the manner in which Miss Davies had carried out her duties as Registrar, and stated that her unfailing devotion to duty, her far-seeing administration of the Council's work and her cheerful determination to surmount all difficulties were deserving of the highest praise"[9]. She had had 25 years' service with the Council, 13 of them as Registrar and a presentation was made.

In January 1948 the Council appointed its first Education Officer—Miss M. Houghton, M.B.E. Miss Houghton, who at the time was a member of Council, trained at King's College Hospital, London, and was at the time of her appointment, Senior Sister Tutor at University College Hospital, London. She was author or joint author of several books in the Nurses Aids series. On taking up her appointment Miss Houghton vacated her seat on the Council.

Also in April 1948, it was reported that the Organisation and Methods Division of the Treasury had carried out an investigation on the work of the Council.

In the Chairman's report in 1950 it was stated that the blast walls (erected at the beginning of the war) had been removed, and all war damage made good.

PERSONALITIES

For the years 1945–1950 the Chairman of Council was Miss D. M. Smith, who in November 1945 was congratulated on her appointment as Matron of Guy's Hospital—she had previously been Matron of the Middlesex Hospital.

The Vice-Chairman in 1945, 1946 and 1947 was Miss M. Jones, O.B.E., A.R.R.C., M.A., and in 1948, 1949 and 1950 was Miss C. H. Alexander.

Once again, during this period, the deaths of several early members and pioneers were reported and tribute paid at Council meetings. In March 1945, Miss M. G. Montgomery died—she had been one of the first two ex-matrons to assist the Council in the 1930s with the inspection of training schools. Also in March the death of Miss S. A. Villiers was announced. She had trained at St. Bartholomew's Hospital and had been a great friend and supporter of Mrs. Fenwick. She was an appointed member of the caretaker Council and was the elected representative of the fever nurses until 1937.

In March 1946, Miss R. Darbyshire, C.B.E., R.R.C., died. She had been Matron of St. Mary's Hospital, London, and University College Hospital, London, was a member of Council from 1933–7 and Vice-Chairman of Council in 1935, 1936 and 1937.

In 1947 Ethel Gordon Fenwick died at the age of 90. Mrs. Fenwick had broken her thigh in June 1946 and after a considerable struggle had agreed to be admitted to St. Bartholomew's Hospital. In November she was moved to the home of a friend and colleague, Mrs. Mabel Barber, S.R.N., R.M.N., D.N., whose husband was the vicar of London Colney, Herts. She died there on March 13th[10].

Tributes to Mrs. Fenwick poured in from the Hon. Secretary of the National Council of Nurses, Miss Lavinia Dock, Miss A. Goodrich and Dean Effie Taylor (eminent nurses in the United States of America); the Nursing Associations of America, Canada, New Zealand, Norway and India; the past-president of the Royal Victorian College of Nursing, Australia, and the editor of the American Journal of Nursing; the Trained Nurses of France, the International Council of Nurses and two members of Parliament[11].

The Council paid tribute at their March meeting, and the press said "The death of a pioneer; she had outstanding ability and was an excellent speaker, a capable organiser and a woman with vision and originality"[12]. The *British Journal of Nursing* spoke of the greatest nurse within living memory, who had laid down the burden of her life.

Mrs. Fenwick's obituary in *The Times* spoke of a woman "lavishly endowed with outstanding gifts of intellect. She devoted her whole life to professional nursing affairs, and among her outstanding achievements was the passing of the Nurses Act of 1919. She was essentially a reformer, dogged and uncompromising and history will no doubt acclaim her as one of the foremost women of her century"[13].

A memorial service was held at St. Bartholomew's Hospital in the church of St. Bartholomew-the-Less, on March 19th.

Years later Dame Ellen Musson said "She felt very strongly that Mrs. Fenwick had not received due recognition in her own country, because Miss Nightingale, still living, overshadowed all others". She (Dame Ellen) felt strongly that we should remember that the work done by Mrs. Fenwick is more realised in other countries than in our own[14].

The authors were both student nurses at the time of Mrs. Fenwick's death and have both always been interested in professional matters, but until recently were unaware of the tremendous part that she played in nursing politics. They find it incredible how little is taught, or remembered, in this country, about a woman who in spite of her obviously difficult personality devoted her whole life—not unsuccessfully—to the nursing profession. No official honour was awarded to her; but perhaps, even if it had been, she would have valued most the fact that she was State Registered Nurse No. 1.

In 1948 the names of the new appointed members of Council were announced. They were:

Ministry of Health:	Mr. S. W. Barnes
	Dr. R. R. Bonford
	Dr. H. M. C. Macaulay ⎫
	Dr. W. Rees Thomas ⎬ re-appointed
	Dame Katherine Watt, ⎭
	D.B.E., R.R.C.
Ministry of Education:	Miss A. Catnach—re-appointed
	Mrs. M. R. Forbes
Privy Council:	Countess of Limerick, D.B.E.— re-appointed
	Mr. John Diamond, M.P.

THE 1950 ELECTION

Although an election was due in 1949, it was not held until 1950 because of the changes in the constitution envisaged in the 1949 Act.

The timing of the election was altered so that the new Council would take up office at the end of September 1950 (not in January as previously).

A complication arose, before the election was actually held, when seven nomination papers were refused by the Returning Officer as the nurses concerned did not, in his view, possess the requisite qualifications.

The 1949 Act was specific in this respect and laid down that the nominee must:

(*a*) Be a State Registered nurse.

(*b*) Be engaged, on the date of the election, in the area for which she (he) is nominated.

(c) Be "engaged in nursing, or in other work for which the employment of a Registered nurse is requisite or for which a Registered nurse is commonly employed".

These essentials were embodied in The Nurses (G.N.C. election scheme) Rules 1950, which came into effect on February 1st, 1950.

As the election scheme was unfamiliar, notices were sent to *The Times*, the *Telegraph*, the *Liverpool Daily Post*, the *Manchester Guardian*, the *Birmingham Post*, the *Yorkshire Post* (Leeds), the *Bristol Press*, the *Western Mail* (Cardiff), the *Glasgow Herald*, *The Scotsman* (Edinburgh) and the *Belfast Telegraph*. The professional journals included were the *Nursing Mirror*, the *Nursing Times*, the *British Journal of Nursing*, *The Hospital and Social Services Journal* and the *Mental Health Services Journal*.

The notice of election fixed 12 noon, March 24th, 1950 as the latest date for the receipt of nomination papers; this allowed 49 clear days (the statutory minimum was 28), in view of the "novelty and comparative complexity" of the new system.

The number of nomination papers received was 197, plus three which arrived too late. The number of persons nominated was as follows:

	Nominations	Rejected	Withdrawn	Remaining
General	132	9	2	121
Mental	17	—	2	15
Sick Children's	2	—	—	2
Total	151	9	4	138

Of those rejected as invalid, two were for defects in the qualifications of the nominators and seven for one or more of the reasons already stated.

Two people stood for both a mental and general seat and they are reckoned as two in the statement.

All seven rejected nominees had a certain amount of correspondence with the Returning Officer and in one case—the only one where the nominee was an existing member of Council —considerable discussion took place.

The seven rejected nominees were:

Miss E. M. Crowthers, General Superintendent, Queens Institute of District Nurses

Miss M. E. Johnston, employed by the Nuffield Provincial Hospitals Trust as administrative assistant in a job analysis of Public Health Nursing

Miss F. C. Norman, Chairman, British Federation of Nurses

Miss E. C. Pearce, writer of modern nursing text books

Mr. Ralph Shipcott, charge nurse

Miss C. M. Stocken, General Secretary, National Association of State Enrolled Nurses

Miss A. Wetherell, retired tutor

Mr. Shipcott, unfortunately, was in the process of changing his post, and when he sent in his nomination form was not working in the area for which he wished to stand. The Returning Officer explained that, as with parliamentary elections, "the date of the election" is taken as the last date for the receipt of nomination papers.

The other six did not satisfy the requirement that "they were engaged in work in the area for which they were nominated".

The Returning Officer saw most of the candidates, one of whom sent in 12 nomination papers with a total 103 nominators. In every case he (the Returning Officer) pointed out that no decision could be given as to whether the nomination could be accepted, until after the time fixed for the final receipt of nomination papers. The decision as to interpretation of the Act rests entirely with the Returning Officer and the Act does not allow for appeals on this particular point.

The ballot papers for the election were issued by May 6th and every person registered on 24th March 1950 received a ballot paper. The papers were returnable by 12 noon, May 30th, 1950. The electorate, according to the Register, was:

General	127,242
Mental	12,492
Sick Children's	5,335

As before mental and sick children's nurses voted only for their own representatives. With the new system, general (now including male and fever nurses) nurses had 14 votes, one for each area.

Of the candidates for the general seats, 108 of the 121 sent policies to the *Nursing Times*. Eleven of the 15 mental nurses, and both the sick children's nurses also sent policies.

The 121 general candidates were distributed as follows:

Newcastle	6
Leeds	4
Sheffield	10
East Anglia	6
North West Metropolitan	12
North East Metropolitan	9
South East Metropolitan	8
South West Metropolitan	13
Oxford	5
South Western	14
Welsh	8
Birmingham	11
Manchester	7
Liverpool	8

The results of the election were announced in July and the successful candidates were:

General			Votes
Newcastle	Miss A. A. Graham	Superintendent Health Visitor	6,767
Leeds	Miss K. A. Raven	Matron, General Infirmary, Leeds	10,971
Sheffield	Miss C. F. S. Bell	Matron, Leicester Royal Infirmary	4,744
E. Anglia	Miss L. J. Ottley	Matron, Addenbrookes Hospital	6,554
N.W. Metrop.	Miss M. J. Marriott	Matron, Middlesex Hospital	7,096
N.E. Metrop.	Miss C. H. Alexander	Matron, The London Hospital	9,220
S.E. Metrop.	Miss D. M. Smith	Matron, Guy's Hospital	11,416
S.W. Metrop.	Miss M. J. Smyth	Matron, St. Thomas's Hospital	8,516

Oxford	Miss D. Baldock	Sister Tutor, Radcliffe Infirmary	9,008
S. Western	Miss N. M. Dixon	Senior Superintendent Home Nursing	5,474
Welsh	Miss J. Todd	Superintendent Nursing Officer and Supervisor of Midwives	5,519
Birmingham	Miss C. A. Smaldon	Matron, Queen Elizabeth Hospital Birmingham	5,351
Manchester	Miss L. G. Duff Grant	Matron, Manchester Royal Infirmary	7,733
Liverpool	Miss M. M. Knox	Superintendent Queens training home	6,122

Mental

Female	Miss M. V. Waters	Sister Tutor, St. Laurence Hospital, Caterham	1,744
Male	Mr. C. Bartlett	Senior Charge Nurse, Moorhaven Hospital, Ivybridge	1,925

Sick Children's

Miss D. A. Lane	Matron, Great Ormond Street Children's Hospital, London	1,791

The Returning Officer's statement contained the information about the rejected nominees, and the following figures:

	General	*Mental*	*Sick Children's*
Valid votes	36,552	5,457	2,519
Invalid votes	1,187	200	37
Received too late	962	73	26

The percentage of the electorate voting can be found in the appendix. (Appendix 6.)

The members appointed in 1948 had a short term of office since the Act reconstituted the composition of the Council. The newly-appointed members were as follows:

Ministry of Health
Miss J. McKinlay Calder, M.B.E., S.R.N.
Mr. P. H. Constable, M.A., F.H.A.
Miss R. B. McK. Darroch, S.R.N.
Mr. V. W. Grosvenor, Ll.B,. J.P.
Miss E. M. Hedges, S.R.N.
Miss D. L. Holland, S.R.N.
Miss M. G. Lawson, M.A., M.B., Ch.B., S.R.N.
Miss F. E. Lillywhite, S.R.N.
Professor R. M. F. Picken, C.B.E.
Dr. D. E. Sands, M.R.C.P., L.R.C.S., D.P.M.
Mr. A. J. Sayer, M.B.E., S.R.N.
Dr. H. G. Trayer, M.B., B.Ch., D.P.H.

Ministry of Education
Miss A. Catnach, B.A.
Mr. J. Ewing, M.A., D.Sc.
Mr. L. Tait, B.A.

Privy Council
Mr. J. Diamond, F.C.A., M.P.
Professor L. M. Penson, Ph.D.

The new Council took up office on September 22nd, 1950; of the 17 elected members, 13 were new. Two of the previously elected members were now appointed; of the 15 remaining appointed members, 13 were new. Out of 34 persons on the new Council, 26 took their seats for the first time. Thirty years after its inception the Council had greater powers, wider representation and a bigger staff, including an Education Officer and a paid inspectorate.

GENERAL DEVELOPMENTS

Hospitals

Whereas in the eighteenth and nineteenth centuries, hundreds of hospitals, of all types had been built, there had been virtually no new building in the first half of the twentieth century.

The Local Government Act 1929 had transferred the control of the Poor Law Hospitals, from over 600 Poor Law Unions, to the local authorities.

The National Health Service Act (1946) transferred control of 1,145 voluntary hospitals, with 90,000 beds and 1,545 municipal hospitals with 390,000 beds to the Minister of Health[15]. A handful of hospitals remained outside the Health Service and are known as the disclaimed hospitals—examples are the Royal Masonic Hospital, London; St. Andrews Hospital, Dollis Hill, London; Cheadle Royal Hospital, Manchester; The Hospital of St. John of God, Richmond, Yorks.; and Providence Hospital, Liverpool.

The 1946 Act divided England and Wales into 14 regions each controlled by a Regional Hospital Board. Each Regional Board set up Hospital Management Committees responsible for the day to day running of one large or several smaller hospitals. Teaching hospitals, both undergraduate and post graduate, were not included in this arrangement and through their Boards of Governors were made directly responsible to the Minister. The Regional Board areas each contained a University town with one or more teaching hospitals. The London area, because of its size, was divided into four Metropolitan Regions.

Conditions in the hospitals varied widely depending on how much money had been contributed in the voluntary hospitals, and in the municipal hospitals on the priority given to them in competition with education, housing and other essential services.

During the war all hospitals had been affected by the tremendous increase in the numbers of service and civilian patients, the development of the Emergency Military Service Hospitals and the sharp rise in the cost of drugs—particularly the discovery of the antibiotics.

Nursing

Many of the changes affecting nursing have already been mentioned. The developments in the hospital service had been followed by an increase in the numbers employed in hospital; in 1921, there were 122,804 full time (equivalent) staff employed and in 1951, 224,616 full time (equivalent) staff[16]. These figures include trained nurses, those in training and other nursing staff.

There had been little change in the distribution of nurses; the well known voluntary hospitals could still rely on sufficient applications from intending student nurses, whereas many municipal hospitals, especially those in less popular areas, had increasing difficulty and relied largely on untrained help. Those with the greatest difficulty were the sanatoria, the mental hospitals and the institutions for the chronic sick. The introduction of national conditions and salaries (Rushcliffe Committee and Whitley Council) had removed one of the incentives which understaffed hospitals had been able to offer—that is, higher salaries and a shorter working week. During the 1939–45 war the Government attempted to redistribute nurses by the Control of Engagement Order (1943), by which all female nurses from 18–40 years of age must, on changing their employment, either undertake further training or work in one of the understaffed areas; this move failed since most nurses chose deliberately to undertake further training, especially midwifery. In 1944 another attempt to direct newly qualified nurses into the less popular fields also failed since again further training was usually chosen[17]. The Minority Report of the Wood Committee, signed by Dr. Cohen saw the only solution as compulsory direction of student and trained nurses but (wisely) no government has ever attempted this.

References

1. *Nursing Times*—23.11.45.
2. Ibid.—24.8.46.
3. The History of Mental Nursing. A. Walk.
4. Nurses Act 1949.
5. Ibid.
6. The Recruitment and Training of Nurses (1947). H.M.S.O.
7. Nurses Act 1949.
8. Ibid.
9. *Nursing Times*—7.12.46.
10. Mrs. Mabel Barber—letter 1967.
11. *British Journal of Nursing*—March 1947.
12. *Nursing Times*—22.3.47.
13. *The Times*—17.3.47.
14. *British Journal of Nursing*—June 1955.
15. The Hospitals, p. 491. Abel Smith.
16. A History of the Nursing Profession, p. 257. Abel Smith.
17. Ibid., p. 178.

Chapter 9

EDUCATION AND EXAMINATIONS, 1951–1965

"That is where the difficulty arises, is it not, that the probationer is both a student and a worker in the hospital and the
claims to some extent conflict?" SELECT COMMITTEE, 1925

The *Lancet* Commission Report, 1932, had said: "In many
hospitals, a sister tutor or matron gives all lectures in preparation for the Preliminary State Examination, the honorary
medical staff lecture, without fee, to second- and third-year
probationers and no properly equipped classrooms are provided. In others, the expenditure on nurse education is significant. For example, at University College Hospital, London,
where over £150 a year is paid in lecture fees to the medical and
surgical staff for lectures to nurses, and three sister tutors are
employed, the cost per nurse is approximately £4 10s. a year or
£13 10s. for three years"[1].

During the 1930s the General Nursing Council's minimum
requirements for lectures for the Preliminary Examination were:

Anatomy	8 lectures
Physiology	8 lectures
Hygiene	6 lectures

and for the Final Examination were:

Medicine	10 lectures
Surgery	10 lectures
Gynaecology	6 lectures

these figures did not include classes and demonstrations in the
theory and practice of nursing.

During the 1930s and 40s, Preliminary Training Schools
became established, other lectures being given at set hours,
which might fall in the student nurses on or off duty. At the
end of the war there was a gradual tendency to increase the
length and content of the Preliminary Training School which
was often regarded as a convenient time in which to complete
the syllabus for the Preliminary State Examination. Progressive

training schools gradually introduced block or study day systems, partly to ease administrative difficulties, partly to include an increasing number of classes and mainly because it was realised that the student nurse could learn better if she were removed from ward responsibilities for the necessary time.

Two events helped to improve the situation. The 1949 Act separated the finance of nurse training from the rest of hospital expenditure, thus allowing (amongst other things) a specific amount to be laid down for lecture fees—and in 1951, the Minister agreed that the detailed syllabuses need no longer appear as Schedules to The Nurses Rules, provided the content followed the broad outlines that appeared in the Schedules. This, for the first time, gave the Education Committee the chance to revise the syllabuses without the cumbersome necessity of legislation.

The 1952 syllabus

The new syllabus of subjects for examination was completed and approved for all types of training except fever. For the first time the syllabuses of subjects and the practical ward chart were separated; previously the latter had been a folded sheet at the back of the syllabus; in 1952 it became a more detailed, stiff-covered book.

There was no drastic change in the form of the syllabus which appeared under similar headings as before, but two new subjects were included in the general and sick children's syllabus—human behaviour in illness and social aspects of disease. The layout was in a new and more up-to-date form and considerably more detail was given.

Council specified the minimum number of class hours in each subject—the total being about 300 hours.

The profession welcomed the syllabus and the opportunity to provide a more relevant and meaningful system of nurse-training. It was the result of several years' work begun in 1946. The first draft was held up to await the report of the Working Party on Recruitment and Training of Nurses (the Wood Report), in 1947 and a second draft submitted to the Minister in 1950, was delayed to await the new Council.

The syllabus was circulated to all training schools in November 1952; its use was permissive at once, but compulsory for all students entering training on or after January 1st, 1954. A guide was also issued and recommendations were given as to the qualifications of teachers and lecturers.

Although the fever training syllabus had not been included in this revision, since in 1951 the whole question of fever training was under consideration, Council decided in 1953 that "since it seems a number of fever hospitals will continue to be used for the treatment of infectious disease" the fever syllabus should be revised in 1954.

The *Nursing Times* editorial on the syllabus and guide said that it might be called the tutors' charter, as it "constantly gives support to educational principles as compared with the training or passive instruction approach". It welcomed the recommendations about the block or study day system which gave freedom to plan the curriculum and correlate theory with practice[2].

Examinations

By 1952 the numbers taking the Council's examinations was increasing and the problem of a sufficient number of examiners arose again. At this time there were 530 nurses and 318 doctors on the Council's panel of examiners and even so, at each practical examination, almost every nurse examiner was required. This obviously imposed a strain on them, and the hospitals where they worked. The greatest shortage was in the field of sick children's and fever examinations.

In 1955, Council decided to publish the figures relating to the examinations in the annual report and this practice has continued. The first figures issued showed that 11,804 entered for the final general examination and 9,785 passed. For the mental examination 801 entered and 716 passed.

In June 1955 a national rail strike added to the examination difficulties but with the help and co-operation of all concerned the results were out on time.

The 1957–8 figures give a good idea of the amount of work dealt with in the examinations department. A total of 44,741 candidates entered for the Council's examinations during that year.

This figure included:

		% pass
Preliminary—Part 1	12,463	
Part 2	10,065	
Parts 1 and 2	7,316	
Final general—female	12,264	85·8
male	471	85·2
Final mental—female	498	76·7
male	490	73·9
Final mental deficiency—female	141	55·5
male	120	52·1
Final sick children—female	702	86·8
Final fever—female	202	79·1
male	9	62·5

In June 1961 there were certain changes in the Preliminary Examination; the practical part of the examination was abolished. In the Part 1 paper, the two sections were replaced by a combined paper, to cover a wider range but requiring less detailed knowledge. In the Part 2 paper, questions of a comprehensive nature were set, which were more in keeping with modern nursing trends. From February 1962, certain parts of the section of the syllabus dealing with human behaviour in illness were included in the Part 2 paper.

In 1961, a Ministry circular H.M. (61) 46 granted special paid leave for nurses and midwives to act as examiners up to a maximum of eight days per year and to retain their fees. At this time, for each examination, the Council needed 180 practical examiners and 500 for marking scripts.

From February 1962 there were changes in the Final General Examination; whereas previously there had been two, 1½-hour papers in the morning on medicine and medical nursing, and surgery, gynaecology and surgical nursing, and a 2½-hour general nursing paper in the afternoon, these were replaced by two papers of 2½ hours each, each with comprehensive questions on all aspects of treatment and nursing care of patients. There were to be seven questions on each paper, of which five had to be answered. Each script was now marked and scrutinised by a nurse and a medical examiner; if they failed to agree a small committee would make the final decision. At the same time there were changes in the practical examination; instead of four candidates being examined at one time by two examiners for one hour, in future only two candidates would be examined at a time. The schedule of practical instruction had to be presented to the examiner who was expected to base some questions on its contents.

Another change was that the examination was now regarded as a whole and candidates who failed in any part had to retake the entire examination.

In November 1965 the Council, with the approval of the Minister, announced a large increase in the examination fees (see Chapter 11).

The 1962 syllabus

During 1960 and 1961 the Education Committee prepared a draft of a syllabus with an entirely "new look". This was linked with forthcoming changes in conditions of approval of training schools and the long awaited re-establishment of a minimum educational standard of entry to training.

It was drawn up by a special sub-committee who co-opted two tutors and two ward sisters. It was approved, experimentally, under Section 12 of the Nurses Act 1957. The reason for this was:

(1) to introduce it as soon as possible,
(2) to allow for amendments to be made before final approval was given and
(3) to allow training schools to apply for approval as and when they wished.

This last was an entirely new procedure; in 1952 the syllabus was permissive at once for anyone who wished to use it; in 1962 every training school wishing to adopt the new syllabus had to submit a detailed scheme of both theoretical and practical training for approval by the General Nursing Council and the appropriate area nurse-training committee. This enabled training schools to investigate and rethink the practical training and, for the first time, in some cases to commit a three-year plan to paper.

The new syllabus did not include the existing Preliminary Examination; the reasons for this were given in the guide which stated, when talking about many existing Preliminary Training Schools, that much of the detail at present learnt in the first twelve weeks was unrelated to the practical nursing care of the patient and was quickly forgotten. Another point criticised was the geographical separation of many Preliminary Training Schools, which resulted in a splitting off of the Introductory Course from the overall teaching programme and the wards. With the new syllabus it was hoped to integrate all subjects throughout training.

The 1962 syllabus has three main sections:
(1) Principles and practice of nursing including first aid.
(2) The study of the human individual.
(3) Concepts of the nature and cause of disease and principles of prevention and treatment.

Training should start with an eight-week introductory course and subsequent theoretical training should be given in a further 14–16 weeks in study days or study blocks; all new material should have been introduced by the fourth month of the third year. Formal lectures should be used only for the introduction of new material and by the medical and specialist staff; every effort should be made "to increase the time spent in clinical teaching, group discussion, seminars and any method of teaching, or use of visual aids, which ensures and encourages the active participation of student nurses in their educational programme". It is advised that tutors resist the temptation to "cover the syllabus".

A separate sheet of paper in the guide gives the suggested minimum class hours which are more flexible than before, to allow training schools to concentrate on their own specialities.

Plans submitted must include those for an Intermediate Examination to be taken within the first 15 months of training; this should include assessment of both ward and school work, and practical ward tests may be observed from time to time by the Council's inspectors.

The record of practical instruction has been altered completely and now allows for far more individual entries by ward sisters and clinical instructors. It is a more practical (pocket) size and plastic covers are available. This ward chart was introduced for all students in 1962 and hospitals did not have to wait for approval in order to use it.

The sick children's training syllabus was revised in the same way in 1964.

The new syllabus was well received by the profession; by 1965 about one-half of the training schools in England and Wales had been approved to use it; by 1967 some three-quarters—and all will need to gain approval during 1968 since the last Preliminary State Examination is to be held in October 1969.

In 1967 the Council asked training schools which had been using the syllabus for several years, for comments; these are being studied and used for a revision.

With the change of syllabuses in all fields of training, the complexities of the examination arrangements increased and at one point in 1967, 14 separate Boards of Examiners were needed to set 14 different papers. This number will decrease when the Preliminary Examination and the "old syllabus" (1952) Final Examinations come to an end.

The educational standard of entry

In the late 1940s the Council approached the National Institute of Industrial Psychology and asked them to design a "test" suitable for entrants to student nurse training; this was to supersede the pre-war Test Examination and would, it was hoped, be used for candidates without School Certificate or its equivalent.

When it was ready, and standardisation tests had been completed, Council approached the Minister (1950) to ask if it could be used. The Minister was unable to agree since he wished to wait for the results of a test being carried out on his behalf by the National Institute.

In February 1952, the Minister wrote to the Council to say that he had studied the Institute's report and felt that he could not approve the re-institution of a Test Educational Examination; he suggested the Council should approach him again in a year, which they did.

In the Council's annual report published in 1953 the following statement appeared: "little was it envisaged when the test was first drawn up by the Institute, in 1948, that the matter would still be unresolved at the end of five years". In March 1954, the third and final report was received from the National Institute by the Council; this completed the experiment which was carried out on some 2,000 student nurses entering training.

The Council felt that the results warranted further trial and again approached the Minister. He felt that methods of selection were best left to the discretion of hospital authorities and thought the test was unsuitable; he agreed to discuss the matter with the Council's representatives. At the meeting, he said that he felt that the results of the experiments with the test did not prove that it would achieve its purpose. However, some progress was being made since the Minister wrote to the Royal College of Nursing asking them to encourage matrons to exercise careful selection of candidates for training. The College wrote to Council asking if training schools and Area Nurse-Training Committees could use the test on a voluntary basis and this was agreed. At this time it was thought that 12 per cent of the total "wastage" of student nurses from training was attributable to lack of education or intellectual ability.

At this time questions were asked in the House of Commons. Mrs. Braddock asked the Parliamentary Secretary to the Minister of Health: "Will the Parliamentary Secretary consult the representatives of the Ministry on the General Nursing Council, because it is becoming the opinion of Hospital Management Committees that the suggested alterations in the regulations for the recruitment of nurses, that are being pressed by the G.N.C., are having a serious effect upon the recruitment of nurses. . . . Had the Minister's attention been drawn to the resolution, approved by the Association of Hospital Management Committees, with reference to the difficulties experienced in recruitment due to the actions by the G.N.C. in endeavouring to raise the present educational entrance examination." Miss Hornsby-Smith replied: "The Minister has received these resolutions; there is no educational entrance examination for student nurses and no such examination can be instituted without the Minister's approval, which he has hitherto refused to give"[3].

During 1955, 1956, and 1957 the Council continued to ask and the Minister continued to say no.

In February 1958 an analysis of the results of 24,500 copies of the test which had been used voluntarily showed that the percentage who discontinued training increased steadily from 5 per cent amongst those who scored A, to 57 per cent amongst those who scored E.

In his report to the Minister for 1958, Sir John Charles, chief medical officer at the Ministry referred to the proposals to re-introduce an educational minimum in an endeavour to eradicate at least one cause of wastage[4].

In March 1960 the Minister finally agreed to an educational entrance test from July 1st, 1962, for those candidates wishing to train for the general and sick children's registers.

In August 1961 there were more questions in the House of Commons which seem to reflect a change in attitude; members were worried about nursing auxiliaries or assistants, who could not speak English, being left in charge of wards, and giving out medicines. Miss Pitt, the Parliamentary Secretary, was able to reassure the House; this did not happen and the situation was improving; as from 1962, student nurses must have an educational standard of entry to include "O" Level English or Welsh!

The Council had asked for a re-introduction of a minimum standard of entry for 16 years. The Nurses Rules Approval Instrument, 1961, stated: "as from the first day of July 1962, an applicant shall not be admitted to a preliminary training school course of an approved training institution for registered general nurses or for registered sick children's nurses, or for registered fever nurses unless:

(a) She holds a General Certificate of Education at Ordinary Level in two subjects of which one shall be English (or Welsh) Language, and she produces evidence that she has completed a full-time course of at least five years in a secondary school or schools, or in a secondary school and an establishment for further education, and that during such a period she has studied and reached a satisfactory standard in at least five additional subjects of general education, or

(b) she holds an equivalent overseas educational certificate acceptable to the Council, or

(c) she has passed Part 1 of the Preliminary Examination, or

(d) she holds such other qualification as may be acceptable to the Council, or

(e) she has passed an educational entrance test set by the Council"[5].

Historians have pointed out that the Act of 1919 was passed at a brief period of time when it seemed there would be enough nurses. It is perhaps worth noting that in 1962, for the first time since 1919, there was a striking increase in the number of young women becoming, or about to become, 18 years of age due to the post war (1939–45) rise in the birth rate (the bulge).

When the educational minimum became compulsory, Council agreed on a pass mark for the Institute's Test; many training schools felt that it had been set too low but they were free to put their own score above the minimum if they so wished. In 1967 it was decided that from July 1st, 1968 the pass mark would be raised for all candidates.

As the original test was unsuitable for overseas candidates the Council asked the Institute to devise a second test for them. This was introduced in 1961; after several years this test was found to be less suitable than had been hoped and after consultation with professional organisations it was agreed that its use should be discontinued from March 31st, 1967.

Age of entry to training

Since the Council's examinations had first been instituted, the minimum age of registration had been 21 years; as a three-year training was specified this in effect made the minimum age of entry 18, but many hospitals had for years accepted candidates at a younger age—sometimes as low as 15½ years. The Council and the profession considered this too young but had no statutory power to stop it. During the 1940s the Minister was asked to permit legislation on this point, and this finally was included in the Rules. On August 1st, 1952, the statutory Rule that the minimum age of entry to training for a student nurse should be 18 became operative.

In the following years, increasing pressure by the employing authorities to lower this age became apparent.

In 1964 Council circularised interested bodies to obtain their views. The Royal College of Nursing, the Association of Hospital Matrons and the Student Nurses' Association all wished to keep the age at 18.

Several Regional Hospital Boards said 17, and the executive of the National Union of Teachers said 18 years for student nurses and 17½ for pupil nurses, provided their work was carefully selected, did not permit night duty for the first few months and included a day release scheme for further education. All the educational bodies approached insisted that there should be no entry to nurse training at an age which would cut short the integrated secondary school syllabus.

In April 1965 the Council issued a statement. Having considered all the views, which had been carefully studied, "after due deliberation, the Council, conscious of the need to provide an adequate and satisfactory nursing service, but bearing in mind that their own prime responsibility lies towards the education and training of the nurse, have decided that there shall be no reduction at the present time in the existing age of entry to nurse training either as a student nurse or as a pupil nurse. This is a matter which will continue to be kept under review". The *Nursing Times* congratulated the Council on having kept its prime responsibility as a statutory body for training so firmly in mind.

In 1966 the *Nursing Mirror* pointed out that "if more attention were paid to avoiding the traumas often inflicted on entry into the profession, the age of entry could be considered in its proper context"[6].

In 1967 the age of entry was one of the points raised by the Prices and Incomes Board when they were considering the whole question of nurse training.

Approval of training schools

In 1949, 878 hospitals were approved by the Council for all forms of training for the Register. By 1957 this number was 958(see Appendix 5(iv)) and difficulties were becoming obvious in the smaller training schools. In the annual report for 1957-8, the Council outlined its future policy; it proposed that in future, from a date to be announced, there should be a minimum of 300 beds in approved training schools, with a daily average occupancy of not less than 250 beds. A wider range of experience would be required and was listed. Council realised that this would result in fewer student nurses being trained in fewer training schools, but it was hoped that the number of pupil nurse training schools—and so pupil nurses—would increase.

At a meeting with the Minister's representatives in June 1958, Council were told that the Minister was in agreement with these proposals.

In March 1959, the Council published its new proposals for the approval of training schools:

(1) A minimum of 300 beds with a daily occupancy of not less than 240 beds.

(2) There must be a casualty department, out-patient clinics and operating theatres.

(3) The hospital, or group of hospitals had to be able to provide nursing experience, in addition to the existing four branches of medicine, surgery, paediatrics, and gynaecology, in ear, nose and throat, ophthalmic, orthopaedic and skin conditions; and in addition one or more specialities of which several were listed.

In the same month the Association of Hospital Management Committees sent a memorandum to the Minister; while they were anxious to co-operate they felt that changes, even if regarded as desirable, would have a disastrous effect on some of the smaller hospitals. They said that the larger schools did not necessarily produce efficient nurses and drew attention to the excellent examination records of some of the smaller hospitals. They did not think the number of beds, or bed occupancy were significant[7].

They urged the Minister to set up a working party to consider the matter and a conference was held in January 1960 at the Ministry.

In May 1960, questions were asked in the House of Commons about the new regulations for approval of training schools, and in the same month, the Central Consultants and Specialists Committee of the British Medical Association gave their opinion; they viewed the new proposals with alarm and felt they would lead to a serious shortage of nurses involving the closing of hospital beds. They considered the proposal to have a 300-bed minimum, too drastic to introduce suddenly.

A *Nursing Times* editorial in June 1960 spoke of the "incredible degree of misunderstanding of the G.N.C.'s policy. Many of the consultants seemed under the impression that it was already happening"[8].

The proposals aroused much interest in the profession; at an open meeting* of the South West Metropolitan Branch of the Royal College of Nursing, 400 arrived to discuss "How shall we implement the new proposals for nurse training". It is noteworthy that there was no speaker from the Council.

* Jan. 1961.

In February 1961, the Specialists' Committee of the B.M.A. passed a resolution that a joint letter on behalf of the B.M.A. and the Association of Hospital Management Committees should be sent to the Minister, expressing concern at the G.N.C.'s proposals.

However, the new rules for approval of training schools were finally implemented on January 1st, 1964. This concluded a long period of negotiation on the age, and educational standard of entry for student nurse training, and the conditions of approval of hospitals in which they were to be trained. An interesting sentence appears in the Council's annual report to the Minister, 1959–60: "a new phase opened on the date the Rule came into operation. . . . Council were released from their obligation to the Minister to maintain an official silence on their future policy, and training schools could review their existing facilities and make their plans to bring these into line with the new conditions by January 1st, 1964".

The fears that all these proposals would reduce the numbers of nurses in training in hospitals were not justified. The number of students entering training remained virtually unchanged from 1962–7 and the numbers of pupils entering training doubled in the same period (see appendix 5(ii)).

In 1962 consideration was given to the Council's policy regarding special training schools which had previously been able to take part in affiliated schemes—i.e. orthopaedic, ophthalmic and chest hospitals. The Area Nurse-Training Committees, the Ministry and the special organisations concerned were consulted and it was decided that specific reductions in general training would be given to persons holding the Orthopaedic Nursing Certificate, the Ophthalmic Nursing Diploma, and the Certificate of the British Tuberculosis Association. A Rule was drafted and came into operation in August 1965.

With the decline of the incidence of infectious diseases, further consideration was given to training for the fever register. The number of students taking this training and the number of training schools involved gradually declined during the 1950s. In the year 1955–6, over 220 candidates entered for the Final Fever Examination from 54 training schools, but by 1959–60 only 170 entered from 29 training schools.

The Education and Examinations Committee met representatives of the Infectious Diseases Hospital Matrons and Nurses Association, the Association of Hospital Matrons, the Society of Medical Officers of Health, the Association of Infectious Diseases Physicians, and members of the Council's own Board of Examiners for the Final Fever Examinations. The views of Area Nurse-Training Committees were also invited and hospitals which had not been inspected for some time were visited.

As a result of these discussions the Council, in 1960, informed the Minister of their views on the future of the part of the register for fever nurses. It was not until November 1961 that an answer was received, which said that the Minister was not yet ready to make a decision. In January 1962 a meeting took place with Ministry representatives. In July 1962 a letter was received stating that the Minister "had decided to make an Order under subsection (1) of Section 8 of the Nurses Act 1957 to the effect that no person should be admitted to the part of the register for fever nurses after December 31st, 1967".

In July 1960 discussions took place about the limited amount of experience available in the field of paediatric nursing. The Education and Examinations Committee met representatives of the British Paediatric Association and the Association of British Paediatric Nurses to discuss the problem. It was suggested that the smaller children's hospitals should consider post-registration courses or combined schemes of training.

In April 1961 a sub-committee, which included a representative from the Enrolled Nurses Committee was set up and further discussions took place. In 1962 draft proposals, based on agreement reached with the bodies mentioned and the Area Nurse-Training Committees, were sent to the Minister. In February 1963 the Registrar and Education Officer went to the Ministry for discussion. Later more statistics were obtained, the proposals amended slightly, and sent back to the Minister.

It was finally agreed that complete training schools for sick children's nurses would need to have a minimum of 150 beds with a daily bed occupancy of not less than 120. In effect this meant that 16 of the 20 hospitals recognised could continue to give three- or four-year training or a post-registration course. The remaining four hospitals would be required to widen the training by secondment. This was to take effect from July 1967.

One of the smaller general training schools to be affected by the 1964 changes in approval was that associated with the Nelson and Wimbledon Hospitals, which were within the jurisdiction of the St. Helier Group Hospital Management Committee. The hospitals had a combined total of 205 beds, including 40 obstetric beds which were not available for training purposes. Following discussion and visits by the Council's Inspectors, the Management Committee were notified that unless changes were made, the Council would withdraw their approval as a student nurse training school.

In April 1962, Council received a copy of a notice of appeal which had been made by the Management Committee to the Lord Chancellor under Section 21 (2) of the Nurses Act 1957. The Lord Chancellor appointed a Tribunal of three members who were: Sir Kenneth O'Connor, K.B.E., M.C., Chairman; Mr. C. W. Flemming, O.B.E., D.M., M.Ch., F.R.C.S.; and Mr. A. P. Babbington, a barrister. The hearing, which was open to the public, was a long one and took place on January 29th, 30th and 31st and February 4th, 7th and 8th, 1963. Mr. R. W. Goff, Q.C., and Mr. Wigglesworth appeared for the Council and Mr. R. Bell, M.P. presented the case for the Management Committee. Each side called witnesses.

In May 1963, Council received the Determination of the Tribunal, which covered 46 foolscap sheets. The Tribunal found that the Council was justified in deciding to withdraw approval in January 1964 if no changes took place before that date; the Lord Chancellor's Tribunal, therefore, upheld the Council's decision.

This was regarded as a test case in view of the 1964 regulations; it was the first time the new appeal machinery, instituted by the 1949 Act, had been used, and the first time in the Council's history that its decisions had been upheld in such a situation.

The Management Committee appealed against the decision in July 1963 but approval was finally withdrawn and the hospitals became a training school for the Roll.

In July 1963 the Education Committee asked Council to consider several matters which had arisen as a result of the appeal. They included the need for closer consultation with interested bodies; the need to ascertain the position regarding the amount of experience available in England and Wales in the nursing of sick children; the need to define the duties of the Enrolled nurse; the need for more statistical data; and the question of the payment of costs. With regard to the need for more statistical data, Council had to point out that such additional work could not possibly be undertaken by the existing staff who were already extremely hard pressed. On the question of the payment of costs, Council agreed that their costs, amounting to £2,864 19s. 9d., should be included in the account submitted to the Minister of Health, in respect of inspection and approval of training schools. The Management Committee paid their own costs.

Nurses in training

The number of student nurses entering training from 1951–65 remained remarkably stable at 18,000–20,000 per year. The factor which continued to cause concern was wastage (discontinuation without completing training) which, although it has shown a slight downward trend is still about 35 per cent (see appendix 5(iii)).

The Council had hoped that the introduction of the minimum educational standard would cause a marked drop in wastage, but this did not occur.

The Council co-operated with the Ministry of Labour in an investigation into recruitment and wastage, using information provided by the Index of student nurses. It covered all student nurses who entered training in 1957, 1958 and 1959, and the report was at last published in 1966. It was a strictly factual survey and contained no suggestions or recommendations as to what steps might be taken to combat wastage. One of the difficulties in any assessment of reasons for discontinuing training is that the main one given is "personal reasons", which as most nurses know may mean one thing to the student, another to the employing authority, and nothing at all to the researcher in the absence of more detailed information.

The Education Department

Once the Education Department had been formed, its staff took over the task of inspecting training schools and advising all concerned on implementing the Council's requirements. By

April 1964 the Inspectorate numbered eight and the post of assistant Education Officer had been created. In 1967 the Ministry agreed to the appointment of a second assistant Education Officer. When making appointments, consideration is given to the applicants' qualifications, so that there are those on the staff qualified to inspect the specialised hospitals—the psychiatric and the paediatric.

Since the introduction of the 1962 syllabus, much time has been spent in helping training schools to gain approval for this. Examination centres are also visited and intermediate assessments are observed. Inspectors aim to visit training schools once every five years but if difficulties arise, or if approval is conditional, the visits may be more frequent.

During the year 1965–6, 117 routine visits were carried out, 26 of these to hospitals undertaking both student and pupil nurse training; 93 discussions were arranged mostly in connection with the 1962 syllabus; and ten examination centres and 13 internal hospital examinations were visited. During the year 35 overseas visitors discussed aspects of training with the Education Officers or with one of the inspectors.

Experimental schemes

Under Section 3 of the 1949 Act the Council was given power to approve experimental schemes of training, subject to the Minister's approval. For the first few years finance for these had to be included in the general allocation, so the scope of such schemes was limited. All the early experimental plans were designed to enable students to cover two or more types of training in a shorter period of time.

For example:

Four-year combined S.R.N./R.S.C.N.

Four-year combined S.R.N./R.M.N.

Combined schemes of varying length to obtain S.R.N./Part 1 Certificate Central Midwives Board/Health Visitors Certificate. Other experimental schemes involved a shorter second training (see appendix 5(vi)).

In the 1960s wider experiments were planned, involving four- to five-year courses including a degree, and shortened courses for the graduate or the candidate with one or more "A" levels.

In 1967 the Ministry announced that an extra allocation of money for experiments would be granted. This was to be linked with the setting up of a research unit at the Council. Meetings have taken place between representatives of the Council and the Ministry to discuss the types of experiments for which financial help will be available. A Research Officer has been appointed.

Some training schools have sought and obtained grants for experiments from interested bodies such as the King Edward Hospital Fund for London, and the Wolfson Foundation. From the Council's annual reports it can be seen that student nurse wastage from experimental schemes of training is persistently lower than from ordinary schemes.

All experimental schemes have to seek re-approval every five years.

Obstetric experience in general training

In March 1959 the Council had discussions with representatives of the Central Midwives Board to explore the possibility of including a period of obstetric nursing experience in the training of all female nurses taking general training. In March 1960 an announcement was made to the effect that the Council hoped to encourage training schools to include a period of two months in obstetric nursing in general training; by October the Council and the C.M.B. had agreed a scheme in principle but this needed a statutory instrument. In May 1961 the Council received copies of the Midwives (Amendment) Rules Approval Instrument 1961 which prescribed the syllabus for a three-month course of instruction in obstetric nursing for student nurses, and made provision for a shortened first period of midwifery training for pupil midwives who were registered on the general part of the Register, and who during the latter part of their training as nurses had attended the prescribed course in obstetric nursing. The instrument came into effect on June 1st. The scheme was permissive and hospitals had to apply to both the Council and the Central Midwives Board.

The obstetric training is popular with student nurses for a variety of reasons including its value when applying for overseas registration; however, it is not offered by all training schools and where schemes do exist the places are not always filled. The Council recognise either gynaecology or obstetrics as compulsory experience and while the latter is considered desirable it is not always possible administratively, since it reduces the number of students available in the general wards of the hospitals.

Pre-nursing courses

During the 1940s the number of pre-nursing courses increased, until in 1951 there were 355. In that year, the Minister of Education was anxious that the number of such courses should increase and the Council drew up a memorandum on their history, purpose and function. The courses continued to be approved and in 1953 the Rules were changed; previously courses had been one year, whole time or two years (four terms) part time; now, three term, part time, courses were approved for certain candidates—i.e. those with two subjects at "O" level, G.C.E., or those who had undertaken a two-term, preparatory course. Candidates had to be 16 by June 30th, before starting the course in September in any year.

In 1954 the Council had discussions with the Ministry of Health, the Ministry of Education, and the Joint Examinations Board of the British Orthopaedic Association, about day release courses.

By 1955 there were 454 courses and approximately 1,000 candidates were admitted each year for training, after taking such a course. In the next few years the number of courses declined slightly but the number of candidates increased. The introduction of the 1962 syllabus, which did not include the Preliminary Examination, involved discussion over the aim of pre-nursing courses, and the Council advised that candidates should take "O" Level Human Biology (or equivalent) instead of Part 1 of the Preliminary Examination.

By 1967 the number of courses was 273; in that year (1966–7) 1,745 candidates entered training having obtained Part 1 at the end of a pre-nursing course and 608 gained exemption from the examination by virtue of holding "O" Level, G.C.E. in a subject approved by the Council for this purpose. It is likely that the Department of Education and Science will recommend a change in the type of syllabus for pre-nursing courses when the Preliminary Examination ceases.

The Platt Committee Report

In the autumn of 1961 the Council of the Royal College of Nursing and the National Council of Nurses (Rcn), set up a committee under the chairmanship of Sir Harry Platt, "to consider the whole field of nurse education and training in the light of developments since the Nursing Reconstruction Committee completed its work and in reference to the part which the nurse is called upon to play in the various spheres of nursing service; and to make recommendations".

The Platt Committee was a large one, with 40 members, including the chairman. They represented nurses, doctors, general and further educationalists and hospital administrators. One member of the General Nursing Council, and its Education Officer served on the committee and another member became an appointed member of Council during the course of its deliberations. The Education Officer resigned from the committee before the report was published.

The Committee met first in 1962 and its report "a reform of nursing education" was published in 1964. The report was divided into three sections:

(1) the case for reform,
(2) the means of reform,
(3) achieving reform.

Many of the recommendations regarding student nurse training were remarkably like those of the Wood Committee Report. The Platt Committee's recommendations included the following: reform was considered a matter of urgency but it was realised that legislation would be necessary; the Committee supported the continuation of the Register and the Roll and the retention by the General Nursing Council of all its existing powers and responsibilities, except for those exercised by the Area Nurse-Training Committees.

Regional Councils for nursing education should be set up to control schools of nursing, which were to be independent of the hospital service. There should be a minimum educational standard of entry for training for the Register of five "O" Level G.C.E. subjects. Students should spend the first two years covering academic study and practical experience and should then take the Final Examination; the third year (pre-Registration) should be full-time service.

For training for the Roll, the Secondary Certificate of Education should be the educational standard of entry and pupils should continue to have a two-year, hospital based, course.

In-service training should be provided for a third grade of ward assistant.

The publication of the report aroused considerable interest and controversy and letters and articles appeared in the press for some months.

In July 1964 the General Nursing Council set up a steering committee to consider the report. It was composed of 12 members from the three training committees (Education and Examinations, Mental Nurses and Enrolled Nurses). After the steering committee had met twice and reported back to the committee, a joint meeting of the training committees was held and an interim report submitted to Council in January 1965. A final report was approved by Council in March 1965 and a memorandum drafted for submission to the Minister of Health. This memorandum was published in October 1965.

The Council did not consider reform as drastic as that envisaged in the Platt report to be either necessary or desirable at that time. They felt some proposals—particularly the educational level of entry—to be unrealistic. They pointed out the efforts made by Council over the past few years to improve nurse education and training:

(a) the re-introduction of the educational minimum;
(b) the introduction of the 1962 syllabus of training;
(c) the implementation of the revised conditions for the approval of training schools;
(d) the efforts to increase the number of suitable tutors;
(e) the raising of the standard of the Council's examinations;
(f) the introduction of clinical instructors;
(g) the continued encouragement of pupil nurse training;
(h) the revision of the pupil nurse training syllabus;
(i) the introduction of pupil nurse training in psychiatric hospitals;
(j) the continued encouragement of experimental schemes of training.

The Mental Nurses Committee found it disturbing that the

whole future of mental nursing seemed to have been based on the proposals for general nursing; it pointed out:

(a) The proposed changes would not provide a larger, or better trained number of mental nurses.

(b) It did not like the idea of central schools.

The memorandum (which was a long one) concluded by stating that "the Council fully appreciated that much thought, based on experience, had been given by those who took part in the deliberations, which led to the publication of the report. They welcomed the attention which had been focused on nurse training and the lively discussions which had taken place throughout the country . . . and were of the opinion that the report would have acted as a spur to the creation of greater safeguards for the training of the student nurse and to the approval of more adequate financial provision for nurse training. Moreover, given careful experimentation and adequate time in which to build up the required numbers of pupil nurses and enrolled nurses, many of the proposals in the report might well in the future be incorporated in a countrywide pattern of nurse training".

The Council's memorandum aroused almost as much feeling amongst those who supported the "Platt" suggestions as the report had done the year before. Just before the memorandum was published, the five-yearly election had been held and not all the newly elected members agreed with it. As the *Nursing Mirror* said:

"When the memorandum was published, a few weeks ago, supporters of Platt reeled under what appeared to be a stunning blow. The General Nursing Council has always taken its history-making responsibilities seriously and slowly and the memorandum had a conclusive ring. Yet only a few weeks later, with the new Council, comes the first whisper of dissenting voices. Already a startling motion has been tabled by six members of the Council, only three of whom are newly elected, that the report published by the previous Council should be reconsidered and the implications of the Platt Report itself should receive reappraisal"[9].

The motion was discussed in camera. Feelings ran high over the Platt Report and one member of the Committee was told by an opposing colleague that she might be forgiven in the next world but it was unlikely she would be forgiven in this one!

In the two years 1965–7 the Council have approved more than one "Platt-type" experimental scheme of training and others may well follow.

TEACHERS OF NURSING

With the passing of the 1949 Nurses Act, money became available for nurse training; this was the first time (apart from the Nightingale Training School) that funds for nurse education had been separated from hospital finance. As a result, many of the deficiencies in schools of nursing came to light and some were remedied.

During the period 1949–65 there was a persistent shortage of qualified tutors and several reports have been published stating reasons for this and suggesting remedies; two were: the function, status and training of Nurse Tutors, H.M.S.O. 1954; and The Nurse Tutor, a new assessment, Rcn 1961.

Where the solutions to problems have lain directly within their power, the Council has sought to improve matters. Their functions, regarding tutors, are approval of the training institution and registration. Difficulties occur because, when qualified, tutors have to work in hospital-based schools of nursing and in this country, in most instances, service still takes precedence over education.

In the 1950s Council recommended that the tutor/student ratio should be increased from one tutor to 50 students to one to 40, and in the 1960s further discussion on this figure took place. It must be remembered that this is a national recommendation, and while it obtains over the country as a whole, it is not true of many individual schools and tutors are unevenly distributed. As with other grades in the total nursing service the picture is obscured by the employment of "other nursing staff"—in this case "unqualified" tutors.

Council continued to inspect and approve institutions for the training of nurse tutors, but many provincial universities found it difficult to attract sufficient candidates. For example, Hull University continued to offer a Sister Tutor Diploma until 1959, when this course ceased through lack of applicants. By 1960

London University was the only one still offering a Diploma course; the three colleges approved to undertake this were:

Battersea Polytechnic
Queen Elizabeth College $\Big\}$ London
Royal College of Nursing

During the 1950s various changes were made, by Council, in the requirements for prospective tutors so far as post-registration experience was concerned. Under The Nurses (Amendment) Rules, 1953, it was a requirement that the experience as a ward sister must be in a ward where student nurses were in training. In 1958, it was decided that candidates must have had at least four years post-registration experience including two years as a ward sister in an approved training school. Special arrangements were made for certain male nurses in the psychiatric field in view of the slower rate of promotion. In 1965, the post-registration requirements were again changed—Nurses (Amendment) Rules 1965—those candidates taking a two-year course were now required to have had two years in a position of responsibility in a hospital approved as a training school for the Register or the Roll, of which one year had to be as a ward sister.

In 1964 the Education and Examinations Committee considered the shortage of tutors and the fact that one of the reasons often given for the lack of candidates was that the available courses were all in London. They, therefore, approached four technical teacher-training colleges, Garnett College, London, and the Colleges in Bolton, Huddersfield and Wolverhampton to see if they were interested in establishing a course for nurse tutors. Bolton College considered that it would be possible to start a one-year nurse-tutor course, in September 1965, at the end of which successful candidates would receive the Teachers Certificate of the University of Manchester. The Council decided that as the course was to be of one year only, a further year's post-registration experience in a post of responsibility would be required for candidates wishing to take this course.

It is too early to assess the success of this course, but some tutors are concerned that the possession of the qualified teachers certificate will not encourage tutors to stay in the hospital schools when salary and conditions are so much more attractive in the colleges of further education. Bolton College has since started a four-term sandwich course for unqualified tutors with several years' teaching experience which will lead to the same qualification.

In 1962, London University published its new regulations for the content of the nurse-tutor course. It was noted that although 275 hours was to be devoted to the basic sciences and 125 hours to the nature of disease, only 25 hours was given to the "development and organisation of the school of nursing". Council expressed its concern to the University but were assured that the training institutions would be allowed considerable flexibility, and the Council would be consulted whenever further revision was contemplated. The revised syllabus came into operation in October 1963.

A welcome development in 1963–4 was the approval by the Minister of the Council's plans for compulsory refresher courses of one week every five years, for nurse tutors. The first one was held in September 1964, at Queen Elizabeth College, London, and these are organised by the Rcn.

For years, tutors had used the letters S.T.D. after their names, to indicate that they possessed the Sister Tutor Diploma; in 1965 London University stated that the use of these letters was not authorised by them and Council agreed that the letters R.N.T. (Registered Nurse Tutor) should be allowed.

Council had realised for years that an anomaly existed in that they could not recognise as registered tutors those qualified teachers who were also nurses. In 1967 the Teachers of Nursing Bill, to amend Section 17 of the Nurses Act 1957, was passed. This allowed Council to recognise "those with such other qualifications for the teaching of nurses as may be prescribed". The Rules subsequently prescribed those who could be registered as Nurse Tutors. It was estimated that this would allow some 30 teachers to register as tutors at once and probably about ten more each year. It was also hoped that it would enable those nurses living away from London, and unable to leave home, to take a local teacher training course if they wished to become tutors.

Clinical instructors

One of the developments in nurse training during the 1960s was the recognition of the need for trained clinical instructors to carry out practical teaching in the ward situation. This became necessary since ward sisters found it increasingly difficult to fulfil their teaching responsibilities, and the tutor/student ratio made it impossible for tutors to spend much time in the wards supervising students in their inter-block periods.

Training institutions such as the Rcn and the King Edward Hospital Fund for London set up courses to train clinical instructors; the Council was allowed a limited amount of money by the Ministry to finance nurses taking these courses and their subsequent employment. On completion of the course, the clinical instructor becomes a member of the staff of the school of nursing.

Much discussion has taken place about the registration of clinical instructors and the Council has approached the Ministry several times on this subject with no success.

Reference has been made throughout this chapter to various Acts of Parliament and for clarity the Acts passed between 1949–67 are listed. They obviously covered many subjects, not all of them directly related to Education and Examinations.

1957 Nurses Act: a consolidation Act which repeated the whole of the 1919 and 1949 Acts and the whole of the 1943 Act except the part concerned with nurses agencies.
1961 Nurses (Amendment) Act.
1964 Nurses Act.
1967 Teachers of Nurses Act.

All these were followed by the drafting and approval of Nurse Rules Approval Instruments, and Orders made by the Minister were published on several occasions.

References

1. The *Lancet* Report 1932. Paragraph 107.
2. *Nursing Times*—20.12.52.
3. Ibid.—15.8.53.
4. Ibid.—20.11.59.
5. The Nurses Rules, Approval Instrument, 1961, Part 3, 9(2).
6. *Nursing Mirror*—September 1966.
7. *Nursing Times*—20.3.59.
8. Ibid.—3.6.60.
9. *Nursing Mirror*—November 1965.

Chapter 10

MENTAL NURSES AND ENROLLED NURSES, 1951–1965

"No man who is correctly informed as to the past will be disposed to take a morose or despondent view of the present."

MACAULAY

MENTAL NURSES

The 1949 Nurses Act set up a Mental Nurses Committee of which the constitution has already been given. At the Council meeting, September 1950, it was announced that The Mental Nurses Committee (Election Scheme) Rules 1950 had been approved by the Minister, and had lain on the table before the House of Commons for 40 days from July 24th.

An election was held for the two mental nurses to serve on the new committee; it was reported in December that Mr. Ernest Dawson, R.M.N., and Mr. Joseph Edward Soley, R.M.N., had been elected; 4,166 valid voting papers had been received and 133 had been invalid.

The members of the committee appointed by the Minister were:

Mr. F. A. W. Craddock, M.B.E., S.R.N., R.M.N.
Miss L. E. Delve, S.R.N., R.M.N.
Miss M. D. Gourdie, S.R.N., R.M.N.
Dr. T. P. Rees, O.B.E., M.D., M.R.C.P., D.P.M.

and those who were also members of Council were:

Mr. Bartlett
Miss Lawson
Dr. Sands
Miss Smith
Miss Smyth
Miss Waters.

Mr. Bartlett was Chairman of the Committee from 1951–5.

The Committee took office on December 2nd, 1950. At that time (March 1951) the numbers in training in mental and mental deficiency hospitals were, respectively:

Mental: 5,083 in 133 hospitals
Mental deficiency: 1,225 in 69 hospitals

From this time forward the new Committee took over the functions of the old standing Committee. The major problems in this field were still poor recruitment and high wastage, and the administrative difficulties caused by the separation of the male and female sides of most hospitals.

Before the Committee took office, in 1950, Council approached the Minister for his views on the position of tutors returning to the mental field, and the possibility of their designation as Mental Health Officers. This was important since their non-classification affected their age of retirement and superannuation benefits.

When the Council took over the examinations and training schools previously approved by the R.M.P.A., it had agreed to recognise the latter "without question" for a period of three years ending January 1st, 1950; following this, hospitals had to meet the Council's requirements for approval. One early difficulty was the need to institute Preliminary Training Schools, which had been compulsory in the general field since January 1947. It was stated in 1951 that an eight-week P.T.S. had now been established in all but one or two of the psychiatric hospitals.

For the three years 1951–4, each annual report stressed the acute shortage of staff in psychiatric hospitals. Council continued to encourage secondment of student nurses from general hospitals and experimental 18-month post-registration schemes in psychiatric hospitals in an effort to lessen this. Both the Council and the Committee felt strongly that shortening the normal period of training was not the answer. In each of the three years the number of those in training decreased slightly.

In 1953 the Minister drew up and published a memorandum suggesting courses of action designed to improve the staff position in mental hospitals and mental deficiency institutions; this was done without any reference to, or discussion with, the Mental Nurses Committee and the Council protested to the Minister. He regretted the Council's concern and said he intended to consult the Mental Nurses Committee before sending advice on specific training questions, mentioned in the memorandum, to hospital authorities. A meeting of representatives of the Minister and the Mental Nurses Committee was subsequently held to discuss the recommendations on the training of nurses made by the Minister's Standing Mental Health Advisory Committee.

The position did not improve greatly and during 1954 questions were asked in the House of Commons, on many occasions, about the failure of recruitment. The following figures are self-evident:

	Mental hospitals	Mental deficiency hospitals
Nos. in training at:		
31.3.51	5,083	1,225
31.3.52	4,614	1,161
31.3.53	4,439	1,080
31.3.54	4,299	1,040
31.3.55	4,103	916

In 1956 it was noted that although the numbers in training were much the same, the numbers passing the Final Examination were slightly improved. The Mental Nurses Committee felt this was partly due to the success of the 18-month post registration schemes of training and withdrew the limitation they had previously imposed on the numbers of hospitals approved to do this. The numbers increased rapidly (see appendix 5 (iv)). The Committee drew the attention of Area Nurse-Training Committees to the fact that they were willing to consider one-year schemes of post registration training for R.M.N.s doing mental deficiency training and vice versa. In the same year the Committee undertook a substantial revision of the syllabuses for examination in both fields and these became operative in 1957.

In the next few years the numbers in training increased—in some cases quite substantially; but at the same time the wastage rate increased to a quite alarming degree.

Mental Hospitals		
Total nos. in training	Nos. entering training	Nos. discontinuing
1957–8	4,877	2,218	1,587
1959–60	6,033	2,620	1,660
1964–5	6,235	2,309	1,428

Mental Subnormality Hospitals

	Total nos. training	Nos. entering training	Nos. discontinuing
1957–8	1,057	526	409
1959–60	1,493	791	451
1964–5	1,695	686	446

1957 syllabus

It will be remembered that mental nurses had never been particularly happy with the Preliminary State Examination, which was taken by nurses training for all parts of the Register. The Mental Nurses Committee also felt that, in the past, training for the mental parts of the Register had followed the pattern of general training too closely. Also tremendous changes had taken place in the attitude to, and the treatment of, the mentally ill which was changing from a custodial to a curative service.

A special sub-committee was set up to revise the syllabuses; in June 1956, Council approved a draft revised syllabus of subjects for examination for the certificate of mental nursing, a guide to the syllabus and an outline plan of training. The documents were sent to interested bodies including the Area Nurse-Training Committees and their comments were invited. In January 1957 the Mental Nurses Committee submitted the amended documents for the approval of Council. Council requested the Minister to approve the syllabus for adoption as an experimental scheme for a period of five years. The Minister's approval was received and the documents circulated to all training schools in March 1957. Training schools had to apply to the Mental Nurses Committee to be approved to use the experimental syllabus.

A similar review of the mental deficiency syllabus took place later in the year.

The new approach inherent in the 1957 syllabus was stated in the preface; two aspects had been borne in mind, one—the modern concept of the mental hospital as a therapeutic community, and the other—the educational principle that learning has more meaning if directly related to the practical situation. The guide pointed out that situation-centred teaching was "the most effective method of ensuring that learning is integrated, understood and retained". It also called for closer links between the school of nursing and the wards and departments of the hospital, which in turn needed the establishment of a Nursing Education Committee to implement the scheme. The composition of this was laid down. Formal classes should be kept to a minimum, discussion and seminars encouraged, and clinical instruction should be the aim of all. The Preliminary Course of instruction should be used to awaken the students' interest and the desire to play a part in solving the problems presented in the care of individuals suffereing from mental illness, and should not be a period into which the whole of the first year's theoretical instruction should be compressed.

The syllabus had three parts: the systematic study of the human individual; the skills required in dealing with mental and physical illness occurring in psychiatric patients; and concepts of mental illness, psychiatry and psychopathology. The press said they hoped the new approach to training "would attract many more men and women specially suited to this work"[1].

The 1957 syllabus for mental nurses obviously led the way to a rethinking of general training and so to the 1962 syllabus.

Changes in the examination system formed part of the new syllabus; it did not include the Preliminary Examination but substituted for it an Intermediate examination, which would grant exemption from the Preliminary examination if a nurse trained in accordance with the 1957 syllabus subsequently trained for admission to any other part of the Register. The reverse was also true. The Intermediate examination was to include a written, oral and practical part and could be taken after the first year of training.

The new Final Examination details were published later. This embodied a structured answer type of question paper; a practical situation was printed; the particular information required was listed as sub-headings and a precise number of lines stated for each answer.

By October 1959 the Mental Nurses Committee decided to abolish the oral and practical parts of the intermediate examination and to introduce a structured answer paper; and from February 1960, the Final Examination was to consist of one three-hour paper, which was to be comprehensive, to replace the existing two papers, and a one-hour combined oral and practical with one medical and two nurse examiners.

By March 1958, 27 mental and 10 mental deficiency hospitals were approved to adopt the new syllabus. The first new Intermediate Examination took place in October 1958.

In May 1964 the Council approved a recommendation of the Mental Nurses Committee to the effect that the 1957 syllabuses, as revised by a sub-committee, should cease to be experimental and should be adopted by all mental hospitals and hospitals for the mentally sub-normal approved as training schools, by January 1st, 1965. At the date on which this decision was made, only three mental hospitals and one hospital for the mentally subnormal were not already approved to train under the experimental syllabus.

The mental and mental subnormality parts of the Register

From the late 1950s onwards it became obvious that some psychiatric nurses were becoming concerned about the future of the special parts of the Register. It is difficult to pinpoint one reason for this and probable that many factors were involved, e.g.:

(a) poor recruitment;

(b) the development of, and plans for, psychiatric units in general hospitals;

(c) the encouragement of comprehensive schemes of training; and

(d) the decision to close the fever register in 1967.

In 1961, questions were asked in the House of Commons and the Minister said the anxiety was groundless.

In view of the concern and widespread, if unfounded, rumours that there were plans for closing the Register, the Council issued a statement in January 1963:

"To allay the disquiet and unrest that have permeated the mental field ever since the Minister of Health made his speech in March 1961 about the future of mental hospitals —there is no present intention to close the part of the Register for mental nurses and for nurses for the mentally subnormal, or to cease to train students for admission to that part of the Register."

The following figures were given: of all hospital beds, 42 per cent were for the mentally sick, but only 10 per cent of student nurses were in training for the mental register (5,685 mental nursing students, 46,443 student nurses for all other parts of the Register).

This statement did little to reassure some mental nurses and the Council's proposals for its reconstitution in 1967, precipitated further unrest. In July 1967 the Council issued a further statement from the Mental Nurses Committee to the nursing press: "that there had been no change in the Committee's policy with regard to the continuation of the parts of the Register for mental nurses and for nurses of the mentally subnormal".

Similar fears have at times been expressed by paediatric nurses.

The educational standard of entry to training

In July 1959 Council received information that the Minister would soon be prepared to give approval to the re-introduction of an educational standard entry to student nurse training. Since the pre-war test had applied equally to all student nurses, and all negotiations with the Minister had discussed "student nurses" with no differentiation, it was with consternation that Council received the news on September 8th, 1959, that the approval would only apply to student nurses entering training for the general part of the Register. Council protested strongly on behalf of the Education and Examinations Committee and the Mental Nurses Committee, since representatives of both had taken part in all discussions.

By October, the Council heard that the Minister was prepared to extend approval to cover students entering sick children's and fever training and would be prepared to encourage the voluntary use of the Council's Test for mental and mental deficiency hospitals. Council again protested strongly and informed the Minister that such differentiation could only have the effect of lowering the status of mental and mental deficiency nursing at a time when every effort was being made to raise this.

However, both that Minister and his successors remained adamant that until an alternative training was available for admission to the Roll, student nurses in mental and mental subnormality nursing would not be required to meet any educational standard laid down by the Council.

Discussions on training for the Roll had in fact been going on for ten years—and the Council had always been willing to approve any hospital which could cover the prescribed syllabus; however, legislation to widen training for the Roll was finally introduced in the Nurses Act 1964. In October 1964 the Minister agreed to notify hospital authorities that the minimum educational standard would apply for students in mental and mental subnormality hospitals, from January 1st, 1966. In the year following this introduction, the numbers of students entering both types of hospitals rose slightly, and by the middle of 1967, 1,000 pupils were in training in psychiatric hospitals.

From 1964 onwards the future policy regarding nurse training had been outlined in annual reports. A sub-committee was set up to study this in the light of the hospital plan.

The sub-committee were convinced that the three-year training for the Register must be continued. In the future this training must be the concern of both mental hospitals, and those general hospitals in which psychiatric units are developed. It was felt that there was a great need to increase the number of Registered Mental Nurses so that both the new units and the existing hospitals could be staffed by those trained in the speciality. Those points were conveyed through the Council to the Ministry officials, who said that the Standing Medical and Nursing Advisory Committees were to study the subject.

In 1965 a draft memorandum from the Ministry was submitted to the Mental Nurses Committee for their comments, before being circulated to hospitals. It stressed the need for psychiatric units to participate fully in the recruitment and training of student mental nurses, in order to help maintain the level of qualified nursing staff; the Minister intended to ask hospitals for regular reports on how they were implementing the recommendations. The Mental Nurses Committee welcomed the memorandum.

The development of training for the Roll in psychiatric hospitals is discussed under the work of the Enrolled Nurses Committee; there is now a joint sub-committee of the Mental Nurses and Enrolled Nurses Committees which deals with this.

Elections

In 1955 and 1960 elections took place for members of the Mental Nurses Committee.

In 1955, Mr. Soley was re-elected and Mr. L. B. Dexter, R.M.N., was elected. In 1960 Mr. Dexter was re-elected and Mr. E. Dawson, R.M.N., was elected.

The Minister's appointed members were:

1955 Mr. W. D. Jones, S.R.N., R.M.N.

    Miss B. A. C. Michell, S.R.N., R.M.N.

    Dr. T. P. Rees, O.B.E., M.D., M.R.C.P., D.P.M.

    Mr. E. T. Rogers, S.R.N., R.M.N.

1960 Miss Michell and Mr. Jones were re-appointed

    Dr. B. Ackner, M.A., M.D., M.R.C.P., D.P.M.

    Mr. N. Barry, S.R.N., R.M.N.

From 1955–65 Miss L. E. Delve, S.R.N., R.M.N., was Chairman. Miss Delve was one of the Minister of Health's appointed members of Council and was a Principal Tutor. In May 1965, Council received her resignation with regret; she was obliged to withdraw from all outside work, owing to shortage of teaching staff at the hospital at which she worked.

At the last election in 1965, there were 17 nominations for the two seats. Those elected were: Mr. A. J. Croney, R.M.N. and Mr. P. J. O'Leary, R.M.N.

The Minister's appointed members in 1965 were:

Mr. N. Barry and Dr. B. Ackner, re-appointed

Miss B. M. Melody, S.R.N., R.M.N.

Mr. J. Fairbank, S.R.N., R.M.N., R.N.T.

The present Chairman of the Mental Nurses Committee is Mr. A. N. S. Marshall, R.N.M.S.

ENROLLED NURSES, 1951–65

By 1951 the Assistant Nurses Committee were considering a review of the conditions of training of pupil-assistant nurses; at that time there were 2,599 pupils in training for the Roll, in 210 hospitals.

The following year changes were made in the written part of the pupil nurses assessment; this had previously been a quiz taken the day before the practical, but now became a written paper with simple questions on practical subjects, to be done in the ward, to avoid the formal atmosphere of the classroom.

From 1949 onwards, enquiries had been received from mental and mental deficiency hospitals about the possibility of training pupil nurses for the Roll. The Council pointed out that, under the Act, there was no provision for special parts of the Roll, as in the Register, but provided either type of hospital could fulfil all the requirements for training, and could cover the syllabus adequately, there was no reason why approval should not be given. In 1953, the first mental hospital was approved as a complete training school for the Roll with three months secondment for experience in the nursing of sick children.

The number of pupil nurses in training continued to rise slowly as did the number of approved hospitals; the Council's inspectors visited about 150 assistant nurse training schools each year and also several assessment centres.

	No. of approved hospitals	No. of pupils in training
1951	210	2,599
1952	285	3,144
1953	335	3,733
1957	459	4,780

(see appendix 5(ii) and 5(v))

In 1953 the Assistant Nurses Committee were invited to reply to a questionnaire on the position of the Enrolled Assistant Nurse in the National Health Service drawn up by the Minister's Standing Nursing Advisory Committee. This included references to the training and examination of pupil assistant nurses and the possibility of part-time training for the Roll. A report was subsequently drawn up by the Standing Nursing Advisory Committee and this was discussed with the Assistant Nurses Committee in May 1954; three main points were discussed:

(1) The Standing Committee suggested that the assessment should be taken after 18 months training and should be followed by six months further experience.

(2) The written examination in the ward situation was felt to be satisfactory but should be kept under review.

(3) Part-time training schemes.

In October 1954 the Assistant Nurses Committee approved the first part time course; instead of the usual two years, the training was for three years; pupils averaged a 32-hour working week, had to spend some time on night duty and attend the whole Preliminary Training School; they might enter for the assessment any time after 18 months ward work. By 1957, 15 part-time schemes had been approved but the Committee felt that not all were entirely satisfactory.

In 1956 the Committee decided that as from 1958 the assessment should only be held twice a year. As with examiners for the Register, there was a shortage of assessors for the Roll; it was hoped that by having two assessments a year instead of three, assessors' travelling time would be lessened and the position whereby, at times, there was only one candidate from a hospital, would be avoided.

In 1956 the Committee approved an experiment at one hospital allowing student and pupil nurses to work together in the same wards and awaited reports with interest.

One point which had always been felt to be a deterrent to recruitment was the use of the term "assistant" nurse. Correspondence took place between the Council and the Ministry in 1958 regarding the possibility of eliminating the word from the legal title but apparently there were difficulties in framing legislation which would sufficiently differentiate between the registered nurse and the enrolled nurse.

In December 1960 the first reading was given to a Bill whose main purpose was the alteration of the title. When the Nurses (Amendment) Act 1961 became law it required amendments to The Nurses Rules and to The Assistant Nurses Rules. Opportunity was taken to consolidate all previous Rules, omitting any which had become obsolete, and in August 1961 The Nurses Rules 1961 and The Enrolled Nurses Rules 1961 came into operation.

The Enrolled Nurses Rules, Approval Instrument, 1961

There were six parts to the Rules and four Schedules. They covered the following subjects:

The formation and maintenance of the Roll, admission to the Roll, the certificate of admission to the Roll, removal from and restoration to the Roll, and the uniform and badge.

In the definition of title the word assistant was not mentioned—the Act having stated that "the Roll of Assistant Nurses shall be known as the Roll of Nurses, and the Assistant Nurses Committee as the Enrolled Nurses Committee"[2].

The fourth schedule of the new Rules described, in detail, the official uniform for the State Enrolled Nurse. The second schedule was the detailed syllabus of training.

In October 1962 the Enrolled Nurses Committee approved alternative plans for part-time training covering 29–32 hours per week for a period of two years nine months—these were sent to Area Nurse-Training Committees and hospitals approved for part-time training.

At the same time, the syllabus was being revised and the Committee considered allowing combined schemes of training for the Roll and the British Tuberculosis Association Thoracic Nursing Certificate. They also considered the possibility of a minimum educational standard of entry to pupil-nurse training, but it was felt that this could not be pressed until a minimum standard was approved for student nurses taking mental or mental subnormality training.

The Roll and psychiatric nurses

The Minister's refusal to allow psychiatric student nurses to have the same educational minimum standard as general students made training for the Roll in psychiatric hospitals an urgent matter.

Consideration had been given to a one-year post-enrolment training in psychiatric nursing for those already enrolled by virtue of training or experience. The Enrolled Nurses Committee decided on the designation S.E.N. (M) or S.E.N. (M.S.) as the case might be. However, in November 1963 the Ministry informed the Council that as there was no provision in the 1957 Act for the maintenance of the Roll in several parts; once a nurse had satisfied the conditions of enrolment and was enrolled, she could not be re-enrolled so long as her name remained on the Roll. A week later a Private Members Bill sponsored by Dame Patricia Hornsby-Smith was introduced into the House of Commons providing for admission to the Roll by virtue of experience in the psychiatric field, but with no provision for establishing separate parts of the Roll. The Minister's letter, and the situation created, caused great concern to both the Mental Nurses and the Enrolled Nurses Committee and uproar in parts of the psychiatric field.

The choice before the Council was either amending legislation to establish separate parts of the Roll, or to limit the period of grace for existing psychiatric assistants; normally the Committees seek the views of professional organisations and interested bodies in a matter of principle of this type, but time was limited as the second reading of the Bill was on January 17th, 1964. Members of the Committee were generally in favour of separate parts of the Roll and wondered if the legislation required could not be included in the new Bill. The Minister was concerned that the subject was controversial, and as the Bill was a Private Members Bill, it might be lost.

There was much discussion as to whether the Bill should proceed in its present form, amendment should be attempted, or the Bill should be withdrawn.

In December the Registrar met Dame Patricia and explained that although the Committees favoured separate parts of the Roll, they did not wish to endanger the Bill in any way since it was essential that pupil nurse training should be started in psychiatric hospitals as soon as possible. Dame Patricia felt that any attempt to redraft the Bill would result in its being lost, and that the details were a matter to be settled between the Council and the Ministry. The Bill went through the Committee stage on March 25th, 1964 and was finally passed unchanged.

The Nurses Act 1964 was short and was "an Act to make further provision concerning the admission of persons to the Roll of Nurses maintained for England and Wales under Section 2 (1) (b) of the Nurses Act 1957". It gave the Council power "to make Rules for the enrolment of persons experienced in psychiatric nursing and persons having other experience of nursing before 1949"[3].

The Rules came into operation on November 30th, 1964, and the Council circulated all interested bodies with a statement that they would now consider applications for enrolment by persons with experience in nursing the mentally ill or mentally subnormal.

Applicants had to be 20 years old, had to have not less than two years full-time (or equivalent part-time) practice under the supervision of Registered mental nurses or Registered nurses of the mentally subnormal in a hospital or institution acceptable to the Council; or not less than five years whole-time practice (or equivalent part-time) under the supervision of Registered mental nurses, or Registered nurses for the mentally subnormal. Ten days after the Roll was opened 1,886 enquiries had been received, 1,768 application forms had been sent out and 78 completed application forms had been returned. By March 31st, 1967, 16,158 persons had been enrolled by virtue of psychiatric nursing experience.

A sub-committee was set up to consider the syllabus of training and examination for pupil nurses in the psychiatric field. Hospitals applied for approval and by March 31st, 1967, over 1,000 pupils were in training in hospitals for the mentally ill and the mentally subnormal.

The revised syllabus of training for all pupil nurses was published in 1964 and was to be compulsory from January 1st, 1966. It had been devised by sub-committees of the Enrolled Nurses and Mental Nurses Committees with co-opted members. A guide was also published and the syllabus was combined with the record of practical instruction. Training schools were encouraged to use the new syllabus as soon as possible. The changes were:

(a) The training now covered the whole two-year period but the syllabus had to be completed before entry to the assessment.

(b) The assessment could not be taken until the pupil had completed 18 months training.

(c) Every pupil nurse had to have the following experience:
six months medical and surgical nursing
three months nursing of long stay patients
eight weeks paediatric experience (this could be arranged in clinics).
It was recommended that departmental experience should also be included. The rest of the practical training could be planned by the individual hospitals but plans had to be sent to and approved by the appropriate committee.

(d) The Preliminary Training School was to be four to five weeks. Except during periods of night duty, formal teaching was to be continued, throughout training, on an average of three hours per week. A sum of £42 per annum was allowed for 12 lectures by medical staff.

(e) On average, the ratio of tutors to pupils should be 1:30.

(f) Confidential ward reports were to be made available to

the assessors; a national ward report form came into being on January 1st, 1965.

The certificate of enrolment would indicate whether enrolment had been obtained by virtue of training or experience in the general nursing field or in the psychiatric nursing field. The Council's own records are in fact kept as if there were two parts to the Roll. Individual hospital authorities must satisfy themselves that the nurse's experience is suitable for the type of post for which he or she applies.

Special consideration had to be given to the practical part of the assessment in psychiatric hospitals as patients were often not in the wards. If little direct patient care was available, the assessment was to be mainly by discussion and questions were based on information prepared by the ward sister and/or charge nurse.

Teachers of pupil nurses

In 1946 the Royal College of Nursing agreed to conduct the first courses for those who were to teach pupil-nurses; these courses were of one month.

In September 1962 it was agreed that these courses should be extended to last six months and when courses for clinical instructors began, some parts of the two courses were given together.

Applicants to the courses had to be experienced ward sisters and on completion of the course they became members of the staff of the school of nursing. In more recent years many pupil nurse teacher posts have been held by registered nurse tutors and where a school is approved to train both student and pupil nurses, the pupil nurse teacher works under the guidance of the principal tutor.

Elections

Elections to the Enrolled Nurses Committee took place every five years with the following results:

1953 Elected: Mr. J. D. Benton, S.E.A.N.
                 Miss M. G. Burns, S.R.N.
                 Mr. F. W. Lane, S.E.A.N.
                 Miss J. P. J. Smith, S.R.N., S.E.A.N.

Appointed by the Minister: Miss M. G. Butcher

1958 Elected: Mr. Benton ⎫
                     Miss Burns ⎬ re-elected
                     Miss J. P. J. Smith ⎭
                     Mrs. E. F. E. Carwood, S.E.A.N.

Appointed: Miss D. North, S.E.A.N.

1963 Elected: Mr. Benton ⎫
                     Miss Burns ⎬ re-elected
                     Miss J. P. J. Smith ⎭
                     Miss D. B. M. Fielder, S.E.N.

Appointed: Miss O. M. Wain, S.R.N.

1968 Elected: Miss J. P. J. Smith, re-elected
                     Mr. G. Edwards, S.R.N., R.M.N.
                     Mr. F. W. Lane, S.E.N.
                     Mr. D. R. Snow, S.R.N., R.M.N., R.N.M.S.

Appointed: Miss M. G. Tucker, S.R.N.

The Chairman of this committee has been as follows:
October 1950 Miss C. H. Alexander
June 1951   Miss M. Lawson
October 1958 Miss A. E. Squibbs
June 1959   Mrs. I. Graham Bryce
June 1960   Miss L. Jones
July 1963   Miss J. E. Clarke
October 1965 Miss M. Gough

In January 1962, the first State Enrolled Nurse was appointed by the Minister of Health to serve as a member of Council; she was Mrs. P. E. Reynolds who was later congratulated by Council when, in the Near Year Honours List 1965, she was appointed a Member of the Order of the British Empire.

In March 1963, Council received a letter from the secretary of the National Association of Enrolled Nurses pointing out that it was possible for all four elected nurses on the Enrolled Nurses Committee to be Registered (not Enrolled) Nurses.

While it was felt that Registered Nurses had a great contribution to make, they were in fact well represented by the members appointed by Council. They asked if Council would consider taking steps first to increase the number of seats open to Enrolled Nurses, and second to ensure that "only Enrolled Nurses with that nursing qualification only" might be elected to these seats. As an election was in progress, the Council could do nothing immediately, but wrote to the Association to say that the matter would be referred to the new Enrolled Nurses Committee; obviously legislation would be required.

In November of that year a meeting took place between members of the Committee and representatives of the National Association of State Enrolled Nurses (N.A.S.E.N.); the Association were concerned that, with the present legislation, it was possible for there to be no State Enrolled Nurse on the Enrolled Nurses Committee. Discussion took place as to the possibility of the Minister appointing two S.E.N.'s, one male and one female, to the Enrolled Nurses Committee. The representatives of N.A.S.E.N. felt they could agree to this as an interim measure, but still wanted to ensure that all the elected members should be S.E.N.s.

In March 1964 Council agreed to make an approach to the Minister to ask if he could appoint three persons, two Enrolled Nurses, one male and one female, and one person whose qualifications would be unspecified. Discussions have continued but no amending legislation has been introduced. The matter has become more complicated in that there is now an obvious need for representation of those Enrolled nurses whose training or experience is in the psychiatric field.

Recent developments have meant that many training schools, general, paediatric, mental and mental subnormality, now successfully offer training for the Register and the Roll. This, of necessity, complicates the work of the three training committees—Education and Examinations, Mental Nurses, and Enrolled Nurses since their work and responsibilities overlap. In March 1966, 13,382 pupil nurses were in training in 785 hospitals (see appendix 5(v).)

References

1. *Nursing Times*—12.4.57.
2. Nurses (Amendment) Act 1961.
3. Nurses Act 1964.

Chapter 11

FINANCE, REGISTRATION AND DISCIPLINE, 1951–1965

"I am apprehensive that such an arrangement might not allow sufficient time for the requisite amount of—something—to turn up."   MR. MICAWBER

FINANCE

The statutory Finance Committee started with a new structure and a new set of problems. The two non-Council members appointed by the Minister were Mr. W. Hayhurst, F.I.M.T.A., R.S.A.A., and Mr. A. L. A. West, F.I.M.T.A., A.H.A. The Committee's work fell into two main parts: first, to oversee the financial aspects of the work of the new Area Nurse-Training Committees and second to control the Council's own finances which were now organised on a different basis.

Area Nurse-Training Committees (A.N.T.C.s)

The order relating to Area Nurse-Training Committees came into operation on March 31st, 1951. There were 14 committees; 10 had 15 members, three of the metropolitan areas had 16, and one metropolitan area had 17. Their composition was as follows:

4 persons appointed by the Regional Hospital Board (including two nurses and one doctor).

1 person appointed by the Board of Governors—except in the Metropolitan regions where:

    (*a*) The N.W. Metropolitan committee had three such persons.

    (*b*) The other committees had two such persons.

5 persons appointed by the General Nursing Council (4 to be nurses)

1 person appointed by the Central Midwives Board (a nurse/midwife).

4 persons appointed by the Minister, two after consultation with local health authorities, one after consultation with the local education authorities and one after consultation with the universities. One of the local health authority representatives should be a nurse[1].

223

The normal term of office for members of A.N.T.C.s was five years, but at first one-third retired in 1954 so that new appointments secured continuity of the committee's work. The A.N.T.C.s could appoint sub-committees as they saw fit.

Since no provision had been made for premises or staff for A.N.T.C.s, they started life in the headquarters building of the Regional Hospital Board and made use of its clerical facilities. In most cases an official of the Board became the secretary of the A.N.T.C., and the A.N.T.C. treasurer is usually the treasurer to the Board.

At a conference in 1950, organised by the Royal College of Nursing the functions of the A.N.T.C.s were discussed; it was pointed out that before 1948, there was simply the General Nursing Council with some 600 training schools; now there was the Council, and 14 A.N.T.C.s each with not more than 40 training schools[2].

The procedure for financing schools of nursing is as follows. Training school authorities prepare estimates in the first few months of each financial year, for the following year; these include estimates for:

salaries of teaching and clerical staff
lecture fees
teaching equipment
textbooks and stationery
travelling expenses and transport.

The estimates do not include capital expenditure for buildings, fixtures, maintenance and repair. In the Council's annual report 1961–2, it is noted that they had again raised with the Minister the question of capital expenditure for nurse-training facilities. "The Nurses Act 1949, having, through faulty drafting, omitted reference to expenditure on nurse training by Regional Hospital Boards". An assurance had been given in 1951 that amending legislation would be forthcoming, but this was apparently too controversial. The estimates are signed by the principal tutor, the matron and the chief lay administrative officer.

These forms are sent to the local A.N.T.C. for consideration; each area committee then prepares a total budget for all the training schools, which must be submitted to Council by September.

The Council's Finance Committee then prepares its own estimates for the whole of England and Wales. This includes not only A.N.T.C. estimates but finance for other matters directly under the control of the Council. This budget is submitted to the Minister by November.

The Ministry officials then consider the budget in relation to the exchequer funds available for the Health Service as a whole —and in January, Council is notified as to what moneys are available for the forthcoming year. The Council adjusts the estimates and allocates a sum to each A.N.T.C., which then decides how to divide this among the training schools in their area.

In recent years all estimates have included a "forward look" which enables the Council to give the Minister a probable forecast of expenditure and new developments.

From the outset the problems of financing a concern from public money became obvious. In the first year (1951–2) a 5 per cent cut was imposed by the Ministry "due to financial circumstances obtaining at the time". Obviously some difficulties were experienced the first time the somewhat cumbersome machinery was used, but these were less than expected.

The sums voted by Parliament for nurse training expenditure each year are as follows:

For 1952–3	£1,526,200	5%	cut on estimates
1953–4	£1,410,000	3%	„ „ „
1954–5	£1,460,000	5·3%	„ „ „
1955–6	£1,441,500	7·29%	„ „ „
1956–7	£1,458,700	7·26%	„ „ „
1957–8	£1,575,300	virtually no reduction	
1958–9	£1,668,300	approximately 3%	cut
1959–60	£1,686,900	„ 2.5%	„
1960–1	£2,035,000	„ 2%	„
1961–2	£2,212,000	„ 1%	„
1962–3	£2,322,000	„ 3%	„
1963–4	£2,603,000	„ 8%	„
1964–5	£3,071,000	„ 6%	„
1965–6	£3,350,000	„ 2%	„

In fairness, it must be remembered that the Treasury regard expenditure as having a normal rate of growth and that, although the estimates have been cut in most years, the amount approved almost always shows an increase on the year before. It should also be remembered that in the 1960s, expenditure on nurse training amounted to about half of one per cent of the total cost of the Health Service.

For the first few years the Council was hampered by persistent underspending in the areas; in 1954–5 this was £160,605. Sensible advice was not always given to the training schools by finance officers who unfortunately sometimes confused their priorities. As late as 1964, a finance officer writing in the nursing press stated, "it is prudent to buy equipment and textbooks later rather than earlier in the year so that if for any unforeseen reason salaries or fees for lectures increase, then the budget may be balanced by curtailing expenditure on equipment and text-books"[3]. This line of thought is not based on fact since if there is a sudden increase in salaries or lecture fees, the Ministry make an appropriate allowance to the Council.

One major difficulty in forecasting requirements is the availability and mobility of teaching staff. A.N.T.C.s must keep sufficient money in reserve to pay staff who may take up appointments during the financial year. When about three-quarters of the year has passed with several vacant posts in the area, the money is redistributed for items under the heading "non-recurring expenditure" such as textbooks and equipment. It is worth noting that estimates are based on the previous number of staff in post over several years and not on establishments; if all established posts were suddenly filled, money would not be available to pay the teaching staff concerned.

In 1952 the Minister agreed that the wages of domestic staff employed in schools of nursing would no longer come within the categories met by nurse training funds; the proviso from then on was that money would be available for staff "solely engaged in duties relating to the training of nurses". In the same year it was agreed that the sum required for nurses training as tutors (and later clinical instructors and teachers of pupil nurses), should be assessed by the Council in the light of known vacancies on courses, and not submitted on area estimates.

In February 1952, a conference was held at 23, Portland Place, London, W.1, for chairmen, treasurers and secretaries of the A.N.T.C.s to discuss the financial procedure and functions of the committees under Section 2 of the Act. Similar conferences for A.N.TC. members have been held at intervals, the last in 1968. The views of A.N.T.C.s are always sought by Council before any decision is reached in respect of matters concerning approval of any training school in the area; the reports of visits by inspectors are also sent to the A.N.T.C.s and a member of the area committee is always invited to be present at the summing-up meeting at the end of an inspection.

In 1954–5, Council received the first request for money to finance a research project to be undertaken by an A.N.T.C. (Oxford) under Section 2 (2) (b) of the Act, relating to training in mental and general hospitals; this request was met, as were others in subsequent years for projects concerned with:

(1) the work of nurses in hospital wards (S.E. Met. A.N.T.C.)
(2) the use of clinical instructors (Sheffield A.N.T.C.)
(3) the reasons for students continuing in training (Oxford A.N.T.C.)
(4) teaching methods in training schools (S.W. Met. A.N.T.C.).

Reports were received on these and many other matters investigated by A.N.T.C.s; including, the Council's examinations, and recruitment (Liverpool); the Preliminary Examination (S.W. Metropolitan); staffing, recruitment and training (Leeds); recruitment and wastage of pupil nurses (East Anglia); the training and status of the S.E.A.N. (Leeds); the training of psychiatric nursing assistants (Wessex).

In many cases reports were circulated to other areas and comments invited; at times, representatives of A.N.T.C.s came to the Council's offices to discuss specific points. The Council has never been in a position to allocate a yearly amount of money for research or investigation, since this would have to be taken from some other necessary item of expenditure; this inevitably means cutting such items as teaching equipment and textbooks since salaries and lecture fees cannot be altered. The Council keeps a certain amount of money each year in a contingency fund for unforeseen new developments.

The Council's own expenditure

Apart from the money received from the Ministry for expenditure on nurse training, the Council's only source of income is fees payable for examinations, registration and enrolment, and receipts from the sale of publications. Following the 1949 Act, the cost of inspection and approval of training schools was chargeable to the Minister or the disclaimed hospitals.

From 1951 onwards, the accounting was complicated by the fact that registration and enrolment fees were only received once for each nurse instead of as a yearly retention fee. These were paid into a consolidated retention fee fund which could only be used for the work of the registration department.

As the numbers entering for the examinations and assessment increased, so the costs of the examination department followed suit and in November 1965 Council announced with regret an increase in the fees for examinations, assessments, registration and enrolment. The Minister's approval was needed for such an increase and these changes were incorporated in The Nurses (Amendment) Rules Approval Instrument 1966, which came into effect on March 28th. This was the first rise in fees for 15 years and the Council's balance sheets proved the necessity. The changes included the following:

	Old fee			New fee		
	£	s.	d.	£	s.	d.
Preliminary Part 1	1	15	0	2	2	0
Part 2	1	15	0	2	2	0
Both Parts	2	12	6	3	3	0
Intermediate (mental)	2	2	0	3	3	0
Final	4	4	0	6	6	0
Pupil assessment	3	3	0	5	5	0
Admission to Register	3	3	0	6	6	0
Admission to Roll	3	3	0	6	6	0
Trained pre-1925 admission to Register	2	12	6	3	3	0
Transfer from list to Register	1	11	6	2	2	0
Transfer from Roll to Register	1	1	0	2	2	0

As the work of the finance department increased and became more complicated the need for the creation of a post of financial administrator became obvious; there had always been an accountant and supporting staff. On June 1st, 1966, Mr. J. P. C. Davis, F.C.A., C.A.(S.R.) was appointed as financial administrator. One of his first major tasks was to cope with the problems resulting from the introduction of the Selective

Employment Tax (S.E.T.). This levy cost the Council about £8,000 per annum and although vigorous efforts were made to gain exemption for the Council, they were unsuccessful. This heavy item of expenditure which could not have been foreseen when the fees were raised, lessened the hoped for improvement in the Council's balance sheet, and in 1966 the deficit for the year was over £41,000.

One costly item is the Council's five-yearly election—and to a lesser extent, the election for the Enrolled Nurses Committee and the Mental Nurses Committee; the 1965 election cost £18,200. Money is set aside each year from income, so that when the quinquennial election occurs the total cost does not fall in that years' budget.

In 1965–6 the Council's office staff numbered over 200 and the expenses of running the office and paying salaries was over £370,000 of which over £200,000 was for salaries and wages (not including S.E.T.). The sources of revenue have been mentioned and in that year were:

(a) Examination and registration fees   approx. £260,000
(b) Interest from investments   ,,   £40,000
(c) Approval of training schools and
     inspections   ,,   £35,000

The Council's staff are not included in the normal Whitley negotiating machinery for salaries and conditions of service and the Council have to negotiate directly with the Ministry when deciding salaries in individual cases.

In 1966 the Council's property was shown at cost as £184,377 and the outgoings on the property were £42,313.

REGISTRATION

The work of the Registration department continued as before but following the 1949 Act, the Register was no longer 'live' since the annual retention fee had ceased. Once a nurse passes her qualifying examination and applies for registration or enrolment her name is placed in the appropriate part of the Register or Roll, "without limit of time" and is only removed if disciplinary action is taken, or amended if the Council is notified of death.

Although the Register is no longer published annually, supplementary lists are printed three times each year, and a kardex for each registered and enrolled nurse is kept in the department. Some 17,000–18,000 names are added during each year.

In recent years the Registration department has been increasingly involved in work required for nurses trained in England and Wales who wish to work overseas.

Throughout the 1950s prolonged discussion took place between Council and the Minister about Section 10 of the 1949 Act. By this the Council were given power to consider applications for admission to the Register from those nurses trained outside the United Kingdom. If the Council were not satisfied that the standard of training undergone met the standard laid down in this country, they could require the applicant to undergo further training and/or take the examination. From the early days of the Council, certain reciprocal arrangements had been in force with parts of the Dominions, but the new branch of the Council's work entailed much care in investigating conditions in other countries and their training schools. Once The Rules framed under the Act had been approved, individual applications from nurses trained abroad, could be received.

The Rules were approved on March 24th, 1950 and in the next year 146 applications were received, of whom 59 nurses could register at once, 58 had to undergo further training ranging from three months to $2\frac{1}{2}$ years and to pass the Final Examinations, 4 were only required to pass the examination, and 10 were required simply to undergo additional training; 15 were found ineligible to receive any concession by virtue of training received in their own country. The 146 applications were from 27 countries.

In 1945 the Minister had opened a list of foreign trained nurses, under the Nurses Regulations 1945, and Council assumed that with the new legislation and their wider powers, the list would be closed. They were concerned since foreign trained nurses on the Minister's list received the same salary and status as a registered nurse, but paid no fees to the Council and were not subject to their disciplinary procedure; in addition the Minister only required evidence of training and no details had to be submitted. Many foreign trained nurses considered unsuitable by the Council were eligible for the Minister's list. The Minister indicated early in 1951 that it was not his intention to close the list at that time; discussions on the subject took place with the professional organisations. In October of that year Council made a strong protest and asked that the latter should be brought to the personal attention of the Minister. At the time it was known that 58 persons had been added to the Minister's list, two of whom would have been ineligible for any concessions by the Council and 56 of whom would have had to do further training.

In 1952 an advisory committee consisting of representatives from the Royal College of Nursing and the National Council of Nurses agreed to restrict its functions to dealing with persons coming to this country for short periods of experience and their admission to the Minister's list. In 1954 the Council learnt with considerable misgiving that this committee would in future deal with all applications for admission to the Minister's list, that its function was limited to assessing the validity of documents and that it had no power to assess the standards of training. In 1956 the advisory committee issued a memorandum recommending that the Minister should be approached to discuss the matter. Finally in 1957 after consultations between representatives of the Council, the advisory committee and the Ministry, it was agreed that the Nurses Regulations should be amended to provide for the closure of the Minister's list; persons trained in foreign countries were to be entitled to describe themselves as "nurse" provided the country in which training was received was indicated (e.g. German nurse). The new regulations came into operation on August 1st. Hospital authorities were informed by the Ministry that nurses not registered or enrolled in either Scotland or England and Wales, could in future only be employed and paid as nursing auxiliaries or nursing assistants.

During this period the numbers of nurses trained abroad who applied for registration was increasing and this trend has continued.

Year	No. of applications	No. accepted immediately	Countries involved
1951	146	59	27
1955	489	321	39
1960	694	464	45
1965	1,341	966	42

In June 1953, the Education Officer visited Nigeria at the invitation of the Board of Governors of University College Hospital, Ibadan, to advise on the development of the nurse-training school; her reports on this and subsequent visits were such that the Council agreed that the standard of training and examination was such as to be acceptable for registration with the Council. Many overseas tours have been undertaken by each of the two Education Officers in an advisory capacity.

As discussed elsewhere, the decline in the amount of infectious disease led to discussions on the cessation of training for the Fever Register. The *Nursing Times* stated that the suggestion was promoted, with support from the Minister of Health, that the qualification for nursing infectious conditions only no longer required recognition as a speciality[4]. This caused some concern in the fever hospitals. However, after much discussion it was decided at a later date to close the Fever Register on December 31st, 1967.

In 1964, concern was felt in the Enrolled Nurses Committee at the increasing number of Registered Fever Nurses, working in general hospitals, who were enquiring as to the possibility of being admitted to the Roll. They were entitled to be paid as enrolled nurses but were graded as nursing auxiliaries. The Enrolled Nurses Rules allow those students who have completed their training or been unsuccessful in the final examination, to enter for the assessment for pupil nurses without further training; however, to widen this to allow Registered Fever Nurses to take the assessment, was thought to be unwise as it would give rise to difficulties. On asking the Ministry's advice, Council were told that the whole question of nurses who were employed in work other than that for which they were qualified was under review. The three training committees finally decided that this was a matter for the Whitley Council.

In July 1961 the Council received a letter from the Ministry of Health to the effect that the Committee of Experts on Public Health of the Council of Europe were considering the whole question of standardisation of nurse training, and it had been decided that a small working party of experts should be convened to decide on minimum standards of training. The Council nominated the Education Officer to serve on this working party and she has attended many meetings.

DISCIPLINE

During the 1950s the Council's disciplinary procedure was carried out as before—that is by the whole Council for registered nurses, and by the Enrolled Nurses Committee for enrolled nurses.

In 1960 a Home Office Committee was set up to consider the procedure of disciplinary tribunals; it was to consider "the desirability of subpoenas being issuable to secure the attendance of witnesses and the production of documents, and in particular the production of evidence obtained by police officers in the course of criminal investigations".

The Council were invited to submit information, and asked their solicitor for advice. After consultation a reply was sent to the Home Office; it seemed that the Council had the right to apply for a subpoena under Order 59, Rule 43 of the Supreme Court, but as there was some doubt, the matter should be borne in mind for subsequent legislation. The Council had experienced no difficulty regarding witnesses, but some Chief Constables were unwilling to supply any additional details beyond the bare facts given in the form of Report of Finding of Guilt.

The report of the Departmental Committee on Powers of Subpoena of Disciplinary Tribunals (the Simonds report) was published and gave the Council power to secure the issue of writs of subpoena and as a corollary to administer oaths to witnesses; these powers were incorporated in the Nurses (Amendment) Act 1961. The Simonds report also recommended that lay tribunals should always be assisted by a legal assessor; the Council's solicitor agreed this might be advisable in some cases, but thought that the Rules should be framed so as to be permissive and not compulsory, since many of the cases heard by the Council had already been proven in a Court of Law and it would seem rather wasteful of time and money. The Ministry officials did not agree and felt a legal assessor should always be present at disciplinary proceedings.

While the new Rules were being discussed the Council reviewed its own disciplinary procedure and after discussions with the legal department of the Ministry of Health, agreed that the Rules should be amended to allow a Disciplinary Committee to be set up, with full powers to remove names from and restore names to the Register; a smaller Investigating Committee was to be set up to undertake the preliminary investigations.

In The Nurses Rules Approval Instrument 1961, Rule 59 (5) and (6) state: "The Disciplinary Committee shall consist of the Chairman of the Council and eleven other members of the Council, other than the Vice-Chairman thereof, at least two of whom shall not be registered nurses; and a quorum shall be six. The Investigating Committee shall consist of the Vice-Chairman of the Council and five other members of the Council, none of whom shall be members of the Disciplinary Committee; and a quorum shall be three"[5].

This method of dealing with disciplinary matters brought the Council into line with the General Medical Council and other professional bodies; another major reason for the change was the increase in the size of the Council since 1919 which made it an unwieldy body for such functions. Another change was that in future all cases—even in the case of imprisonment—would be investigated fully.

In 1961 the Ministry sent a circular to hospital authorities asking them to notify statutory bodies in all cases of dismissal or resignation of staff concerned with convictions in the Courts. They were also free to submit the circumstances of dismissal or resignation to the appropriate body, even though there had been no conviction in the courts.

The new Rules came into operation in August 1961 and the first meeting of the new Disciplinary Committee took place in October 1961. The General Nursing Council Disciplinary Proceedings (Legal Assessor) Rules, 1961, made by the Lord Chancellor, under Section 10 of the Nurses (Amendment) Act, came into operation on September 1st, 1961. In December, Lord Meston accepted appointment as the Council's Legal Assessor.

In the first few months of their existence, the new committees discussed the problem of nurses, who, when in magistrates' courts, charged with minor offences, were often advised to plead guilty, not realising that the case would then automatically be referred to the Council. The Home Office was notified of the difficulty. At much the same time concern was expressed about the increasing number of cases relating to the misappropration of drugs by nurses. Letters were sent by Council to the Association of Hospital Matrons, the Mental Hospitals Matrons Association and the National Association of Chief Male Nurses, asking them to draw the attention of their staffs to the serious consequence of such action even when quite a small amount of drugs was involved.

During 1962 Council agreed with the Ministry that in future they (the Council) would inform the employing authority when a nurse's name was removed from the Register or Roll, provided she was employed in duties requiring her to be a nurse. When the facts of the nurse's employment could not be ascertained, the Ministry would be informed.

In 1963, Council still felt concern about the number of nurses who were still being advised to plead guilty in the courts. The Council had written to the Home Secretary, to the Association of Chief Police Officers and to the Magistrates' Association, all of whom felt that no advantage would result from meetings or discussions. They advised that it was essentially a matter in which the Council should take action to safeguard the interests of nurses. At the September meeting the Disciplinary Committee considered a pamphlet issued by the General Medical Council to newly qualified doctors relating to the Functions, Procedure and Disciplinary Jurisdiction of that Council. It was agreed that a similar pamphlet should be drafted for issue to newly registered and enrolled nurses. Council approved the draft in January 1964 and the document is now sent to every nurse who registers or enrols.

In March 1964 the Council learned with regret of the death of Mr. S. Hewitt Pitt who had been the Council's solicitor from 1933 to 1959 and who was the son of the Council's first solicitor. The present solicitor is Mr. Hewitt Pitt's cousin, Mr. Walter S. Pitt.

During 1964 discussion took place between the Council and the Ministry as to which disciplinary cases, resulting in a nurse's name being removed from the Register or the Roll, should be reported to the Ministry. The latter had asked that the names of all nurses removed for theft, drug-taking, sexual misbehaviour or any other offence which might directly affect the patient, should be sent to them. The Disciplinary and Enrolled Nurses Committees agreed to notify the Ministry only of those nurses whose names were removed, who in their opinion could be a possible danger to patients, and who should not be allowed to work in contact with patients now and in the foreseeable future. In such cases the person concerned would be notified of this procedure.

In 1965 the relevant committees expressed their concern to Council that many nurses who appeared before them lacked the support of their employing authorities. It was agreed that when a nurse is informed that disciplinary proceedings are to be taken against her, she should be told that it would be helpful if she produced testimonials from her employers. The Ministry were asked for their help in this matter and in July 1966 they sent a letter to all hospitals and local authorities, drawing their attention to this point. Council also wrote to the Association of Hospital Matrons.

The present disciplinary procedure

Council have power to take disciplinary action against registered or enrolled nurses if it is brought to their attention by the Courts, employing authorities or individuals, that a nurse is guilty of a felony, a misdemeanour or of any misconduct which warrants consideration.

In the case of a registered nurse, she is invited to submit a written statement to the Investigating Committee; if the offence is considered to be sufficiently serious the nurse is notified that she will be required to attend the hearing of her case at the next meeting of the Disciplinary Committee, so that they may consider what action should be taken.

In the case of an enrolled nurse a similar procedure is followed but the Enrolled Nurses Committee deal with both the investigation and the hearing.

The hearings are open to the public; witnesses may be subpoenaed and evidence can be given on oath. The nurse may be represented by Counsel, a solicitor or a friend and is invited to submit medical or other evidence of mitigating circumstances. The case can be heard in the nurse's absence if she fails to attend, but if the reason for this is illness, the hearing is deferred until she is well.

After hearing all the facts of the case the Committee deliberate in camera.

There are three possible courses of action:

(a) The nurse's name may be removed from the Register or the Roll.

(b) Judgement may be postponed for a specified period of time.

(c) The case may be dismissed, either with or without a caution.

The booklet issued by the Council contains the following important information:

"The Disciplinary Committee and the Enrolled Nurses Committee are bound by law to accept a conviction as conclusive evidence that the nurse was in fact guilty of the offence; it is not open to a nurse to contend at the hearing before the Committee that she was in fact innocent of the offence of which she was convicted, or that she was convicted only because she had pleaded guilty in order to avoid publicity or for some other reason."

Even if a nurse receives a conditional discharge, the Committees have power to consider the case and the nurse cannot plead innocence.

One of the offences frequently before the Committees is the misappropriation of drugs.

If a nurse's name is removed from the Register or Roll, she may apply for restoration at a later date, but she must submit names of referees who are aware of the reason for which her name was removed. In a case of postponed judgement, the same applies, at the end of the stated period.

Any nurse may appeal to the High Court against the Committees decision.

Another side of the work of the Committees is to take action against anyone falsely claiming to be a "Nurse"—that is without being registered or enrolled.

The following figures indicate the increase in the work of the committees.

	No. of cases	No. removed	No. postponed	No. restored
1956 Registered	18	8	10	5
Enrolled	3	2	1	2

		No. of cases	No. removed	No. postponed	No. restored
1961	Registered	41	14	23	3
	Enrolled	7	4	3	1
1966	Registered	74	17	43	13
	Enrolled	19	6	8	—

With the setting up of the Investigating and Disciplinary Committees, the amount of work to be covered at the meeting of the whole Council was considerably lessened. Council therefore decided that their meetings would in future take place every two months instead of every month.

References

1. *Nursing Times*—24.5.52.
2. Ibid.—8.7.50.
3. Ibid—3.1.64.
4. Ibid.—2.12.54.
5. The Nurses Rules, Approval Instrument, 1961.

Chapter 12

PERSONALITIES AND ELECTIONS, 1951–1965

"Who knows whether the best of men be known, or whether
there be not more remarkable persons forgot than any that stand
remembered in the known account of time."

SIR THOMAS BROWNE

Miss M. Houghton, M.B.E., S.R.N., was the Council's first
Education Officer and held the post for 11½ years; she retired
on September 30th, 1959 and tributes were paid to her work at
the June Council meeting. She had by then given 44 years' un-
broken service to the nursing profession and had made many
contributions to nurse education and training in countries other
than England and Wales. During the 1950s she was granted
special leave on several occasions to advise governments overseas on the development of their own training programmes.
The Chairman spoke of "the important and valuable contribution Miss Houghton had made towards raising the standard of
nurse training and thus the nursing care of the patient". On her
retirement Miss Houghton was asked to undertake certain *ad
hoc* tasks for the Council which took fifteen months. In the 1962
New Year Honours List Miss Houghton was made an officer
of the Order of the British Empire. (See page 244).

The new Education Officer was Miss B. N. Fawkes, S.R.N.,
S.C.M., D.N.(Lond.), S.T.D., B.Sc.(Columbia University).
Miss Fawkes trained at the Middlesex Hospital and had been
Principal Tutor there from 1947–56; in 1952 she was awarded a
British Red Cross Society scholarship to study nursing educa-
tion and administration at Columbia University. She became
an Inspector of Training Schools in 1956.

In 1961 work commenced on adding fifth and sixth floors
to the Council's offices at 23, Portland Place, London, W.1, and
by July 1962 this had been completed. The new floors were
occupied and alterations were then made to the second, third
and fourth floors; when all the work was finished, the staff
working at 17, Portland Place were able to move into the main
building. One room, on the ground floor of No. 17, was furn-
ished for use as a committee room, and the second, third and
fourth floors let to tenants; these included, the National
Association for Mental Health, the Association of Hospital

Matrons, the Guild of St. Barnabas for Nurses, the 1930 Fund, and a firm of chartered accountants.

Members of Council

It often happens that only one person is nominated to serve as Chairman or Vice-Chairman of Council; when this happens, there is naturally no ballot.

However, in September 1960 there were two nominations* for Chairman and as each nominee received an equal number of votes from those members present it was decided to hold a postal ballot so that those not able to be present at the Council meeting could take part in voting.

In September 1962 there were four nominations† for Vice-Chairman and in accordance with the Council's practice, three separate ballots were held, the person with the least number of votes being eliminated on each occasion.

In September 1965 there were two nominations‡ for Vice-Chairman.

The Chairman of Council from 1951–5 was Miss D. M. Smith, who in June 1953 was awarded a C.B.E. in the Coronation Honours List.

The Chairman from 1955–60 was Miss M. J. Smyth who was awarded an O.B.E. in 1955 and a C.B.E. in June 1959.

The Chairman from 1960–5 was Miss C. A. Smaldon who received a C.B.E. in the Birthday Honours List in June 1964.

The Vice-Chairman from 1951–5 was Miss M. J. Smyth; from 1955–62 was Miss J. M. Loveridge; and from 1962 onwards was Miss R. A. Hone. Miss Hone, who is Principal Tutor of St. Thomas's Hospital, London, is the first nurse, who is not a matron, to hold office as either Chairman or Vice-Chairman.

In September 1955, Miss D. Holland, Principal Tutor, Guy's Hospital, London, was elected Chairman of the Education and Examinations Committee; Miss Holland had been a member of Council from 1945–53 and was again elected in September 1955. Although it would seem logical for a nurse tutor to be chairman of this committee it apparently caused some comment; however, the practice has continued ever since.

In 1953 the appointed members of Council were announced:

* 1960—Miss M. Marriott and Miss C. A. Smaldon.
† 1962—Miss J. Clark; Miss R. Hone; Miss M. Marriott; Miss. G. Watts.
‡ 1965—Miss E. Bendall and Miss R. Hone.

Minister of Health

Miss F. E. Lillywhite, S.R.N.
Miss E. K. Trillwood, S.R.N.
Miss R. B. McK. Darroch, S.R.N.
Miss L. E. Delve, S.R.N., R.M.N.
Mr. A. J. Sayer, M.B.E., S.R.N.
Miss E. M. Hedges, S.R.N.
Mr. P. H. Constable, M.A., F.H.A.
Mr. V. W. Grosvenor, Ll.B., J.P.
Dr. A. Walk, M.D., D.P.M.
Sir Allen Daley, B.Sc., D.P.H., F.R.C.P.
Dr. H. G. Trayer, M.B., B.Ch., D.P.H.
Miss M. G. Lawson, O.B.E., M.A., M.B., Ch.B., S.R.N., D.N.

Minister of Education

Miss A. Catnach, C.B.E, B.A.
Dr. J. Ewing, M.A., D.S.C.
Mr. D. C. A. Ker, B.Com., B.Sc.

Privy Council

Professor J. Whillis, M.D., M.S., F.R.C.S.
Mr. W. G. Campbell, B.A., F.C.A.

Seven of the appointed members were new.

In 1958 they were:

Minister of Health

Miss D. J. Berry, S.R.N.
Mr. P. H. Constable
Miss L. E. Delve
Dr. J. Douglas, M.D., D.P.H.
Mr. J. B. Hume, M.S., F.R.C.S.
Ald. E. C. Hutchins
Miss S. Moore, S.R.N.
Miss l. H. Morris, S.R.N.
Miss E. Robinson, S.R.N.
Mr. A. J. Sayer
Miss F. I. Tennant, S.R.N.
Dr. A. Walk

Minister of Education
>Mrs. E. Evans, B.Sc.
>Mrs. I. Graham-Bryce, M.A., J.P.
>Mr. D. C. A. Ker

Privy Council
>Mr. J. S. Fulton, M.A.
>Major S. Whitbread

In 1963 they were:

Minister of Health
>Mr. R. M. Bompas, A.C.I.S., F.H.A.
>Miss L. E. Delve
>Dr. J. Douglas
>Mr. A. Stavely Gough, F.R.C.S.
>Mrs. V. M. John, S.R.N.
>Miss V. M. King, S.R.N.
>Mr. F. S. Lawlor, S.R.N.
>Mr. A. V. Martin, C.B.E.
>Miss A. G. Notman, S.R.N., R.S.C.N.
>Mrs. P. E. Reynolds, S.E.N.
>Miss E. Robinson
>Dr. A. Walk
>Miss D. M. White, S.R.N.

At this time the Minister's appointed members were increased by one since the elected members had increased owing to the division of the South West Metropolitan Region into two, which created the new Region of Wessex.

Minister of Education
>Mrs. V. B. Chambers, Ph.D., J.P.
>Mrs. E. Evans
>Mr. Emlyn Jones, M.Sc., F.R.I.C.

Privy Council
>Dr. Brynmor Jones, Ph.D., Ms.D.
>Major S. Whitbread

Throughout the Council's history some appointed members found themselves, at times, unable to attend sufficient meetings because of their other commitments. In this case the appropriate body nominated another person to fill the vacancy for the remainder of the term of office (see appendix 1(i) for full list).

On November 7th, 1960 Dame Ellen Musson, D.B.E., R.R.C., LL.D., S.R.N., died at the age of 93. Dame Ellen trained at St. Bartholomew's Hospital, London, from 1895–8 and was awarded a gold medal. After being night sister, ward sister and assistant matron in her training school, she became matron of the Swansea General and Eye Hospital in 1906; in 1909 she became matron of Birmingham General Hospital and held this post until 1923, when she resigned on becoming a member of the General Nursing Council. She was Chairman from 1926–43 and Vice-Chairman from 1943–4. She was made a C.B.E. in 1928 and a D.B.E. in 1939; she was awarded the R.R.C. in 1961, an honorary degree of Doctor of Laws in 1932 and the Florence Nightingale International Medal in 1939.

In 1955 Dame Laura Knight painted her portrait which now hangs in the Council chamber.

A memorial service organised by the Royal College of Nursing was held on November 24th in All Souls' Church, Langham Place, London, W.1. The church was packed, and the congregation included representatives from all the nursing organisations as well as from many hospitals and the University of Leeds. A tribute was spoken by Miss D. C. Bridges, C.B.E., and the lesson read by Miss Loveridge, Matron of St. Bartholomew's Hospital. The Council were represented by the three subsequent chairman of Council, Miss D. M. Smith, Miss M. J. Smyth and Miss C. A. Smaldon, together with Miss G. E. Davies (former Registrar), Miss M. Henry (present Registrar), and several members of Council.

Tributes were paid at the November Council meeting.

Other well-known members of Council and its staff who died during this period were: Miss M. A. Gullan (1958), Dame Katharine Watt (1963) formally Chief Nursing Officer to the Ministry of Health*; Mr. A. L. A. West, F.H.A., one of the first two appointed members to the Finance Committee (1966) who had served since 1950; and Miss E. A. Rutter, first Assistant Registrar from 1950–60 (1961). Miss Rutter had resigned in April 1960, because of ill health and died in February 1961.

* Miss H. Day, C.B.E., died in June 1968.

In the *Nursing Times* of February 9th, 1968, two appreciations appeared: Marjorie Houghton, O.B.E., the Council's first Education Officer, had died in Kenya on February 3rd, and as one writer said, "her contribution was not only to nurse education but to the profession as a whole". Miss Houghton, who had retired from the Council's staff in 1959, had had a long and varied career in nursing; as senior sister tutor at University College Hospital she had introduced the first "block system" in the country and as Education Officer to the Council, her ideas and planning lay behind much of the revision of all the syllabuses from 1957–62, and the other changes in training which went with these. One appreciation included the words: "her friends are legion and scattered throughout the world and they will think with nothing but gratitude of a life so fully lived and so wholly enjoyed". A memorial service was held.

THE ELECTIONS

In accordance with the terms of the Act, quinquennial elections were held in 1955, 1960 and 1965.

In 1955, 54 candidates stood for the 14 general seats, 3 for the female mental nurse's seat, 10 for the male mental nurse's seat and 2 for the sick children's nurse's seat. Most of the candidates sent policies to the *Nursing Times*.

The returning officer reported that over 15,000 ballot papers were returned to the office because of obsolete address (7–8 per cent of the electorate). This was obviously due to the fact that there had not been a "live" Register for five years; there was also an increase in the number of voters who failed to sign the identification required on the ballot envelope.

For the general register the number of voting papers assumed to be delivered was 156,348; the valid voting papers received were 45,692; invalid votes were 1,499 and those received too late were 478. For the mental register the figures were:

Delivered: 19,552.   Valid votes: 6,519

For the sick children's register the figures were:

Delivered: 7,421   Valid votes: 3,042

The elected general nurses were:

Area	Name	Post held
Newcastle	Miss A. Y. Sanderson	Health Visitor Tutor

Leeds	Miss K. A. Raven	Matron, Leeds Gen. Infirmary
Sheffield	Miss J. B. Price	Principal, United Sheffield Hospitals School of Nursing
East Anglia	Miss L. J. Ottley	Matron, Addenbrookes Hospital
N.W. Metropolitan	Miss M. J. Marriott	Matron, Middlesex Hospital
N.E. Metropolitan	Miss J. M. Loveridge	Matron, St. Bartholomew's Hospital
S.E. Metropolitan	Miss D. L. Holland	Principal Tutor, Guy's Hospital
S.W. Metropolitan	Miss M. J. Smyth	Matron, St. Thomas's Hospital
Oxford	Miss E. M. Powell	Matron, Wingfield Morris Orthopaedic Hospital
South Western	Miss E. M. Bryant	Superintendent, Maternity and District Nursing Association
Wales	Miss S. C. Bovill	Matron, Cardiff Royal Infirmary
Birmingham	Miss C. A. Smaldon	Matron, Queen Elizabeth Hospital, Birmingham
Manchester	Miss L. Jones	County Superintendent, Dist. Nurses, Preston
Liverpool	Miss K. I. Cawood	Matron, Alder Hey Hospital, Liverpool

Five of these members were re-elected and nine were new. Those elected by mental nurses were:

Mr. C. Bartlett ⎫
Miss W. V. Waters ⎬ re-elected

Elected by registered sick children's nurses:

Miss G. M. Kirby, S.R.N., R.S.C.N., Matron, The Hospital for Sick Children, Great Ormond Street, London, W.C.1.

In November 1958, Council were informed by the Minister of his intention to set up a fifteenth area nurse-training committee when the fifteenth Regional Hospital Board (Wessex) was set up in 1959.

Council replied, thanking the Minister, and pointing out that his letter and the wording of the 1957 Act would seem to indicate that there should then be a fifteenth elected general nurse. This obviously required amending legislation. The Minister replied that if legislation were not introduced in time for the 1960 election it was proposed to designate the areas of the South West Metropolitan R.H.B. and the Wessex R.H.B. as a single constituency. The Council did not regard this as acceptable, and felt the profession would not be happy about the proposals for the 1960 election. A personal interview with the Minister was sought; he felt no useful purpose would be served and could not promise amending legislation. After further discussion Council decided they could not take any action.

In March 1959 the Minister wrote saying he hoped opportunity would arise soon for amending legislation but nothing further was done in time for the election. The changes were finally incorporated in the Nurses (Amendment) Act 1961 which provided for two extra members—one to be elected for the Wessex Area, and one appointed.

In 1960, 53 candidates stood for the 14 general seats, 9 for the male mental nurse's seat, 3 for the female mental nurse's seat and 1 for the sick children's representative who was declared elected, unopposed.

The returning officer stated that it was assumed that 217,430 voting papers had been received and a large number were returned undelivered. He stated that from the percentage who voted it seemed there was less interest than in the 1955 election; the percentage voting was 25·46 as compared with 31·26 in 1955.

Those elected for the 14 general seats were:

Area	Name	Post held
Newcastle	Miss F. Shaw	Matron, Royal Victoria Infirmary, Newcastle
Leeds	Miss G. E. Watts	Matron, The General Infirmary, Leeds
Sheffield	Miss P. Goodall	Principal Tutor, Leicester Royal Infirmary
East Anglia	Miss K. M. Allison	Matron, West Norfolk and King's Lynn General Hospital
N.W. Metropolitan	Miss M. J. Marriott	Matron, The Middlesex Hospital, London
N.E. Metropolitan	Miss J. M. Loveridge	Matron, St. Bartholomew's Hospital, London
S.E. Metropolitan	Miss J. E. Clark	Regional Nursing Officer
S.W. Metropolitan	Miss R. A. Hone	Principal Tutor, St. Thomas's Hospital, London
Oxford	Miss E. Preddy	Matron, United Oxford Hospitals
South Western	Miss R. M. Furze	Matron, Royal Devon and Exeter Hospital
Wales	Miss M. A. Gough	Principal Tutor, Cardiff Royal Infirmary

Birmingham	Miss C. A. Smaldon	Chief Nursing Officer, United Birmingham Hospitals
Manchester	Miss L. Jones	Superintendent of District Nurses, Lancashire County Council
Liverpool	Miss K. I. Cawood	Matron, Alder Hey Hospital, Liverpool

Of these, four were re-elected and ten were new.

Those elected by mental nurses were:

Mrs. E. C. Knowles, Ward Sister, Forest Hospital, Horsham
Mr. J. E. Soley, Deputy Chief Male Nurse, Goodmayes Hospital, Essex.

Both members were new.

Elected by sick children's nurses:

Miss G. M. Kirby, re-elected unopposed.

The 1965 election evoked even less interest than that held in 1960 and this trend was particularly obvious in the number of candidates standing for election. The regional pattern was as follows:

General candidates:

Newcastle	One candidate
Leeds	Two candidates
Sheffield	Two candidates
East Anglia	Three candidates
North West Metropolitan	Two candidates
North East Metropolitan	Two candidates
South East Metropolitan	Two candidates
South West Metropolitan	One candidate
Oxford	Two candidates
South Western	One candidate
Wales	One candidate
Birmingham	Two candidates
Manchester	Two candidates
Liverpool	No candidate
Wessex	Three candidates

Mental nurses
   Male nurse, 13 candidates
   Female nurse, 3 candidates

Sick children's nurses
   One candidate

As the press pointed out, it was a disappointing response to an expensive undertaking; in five cases, candidates were unopposed and no election could be held and in one region no-one had been nominated at all. They also commented on the marked decrease in the number of matrons standing for election and the marked increase in the number of tutors.

Nearly 67,000 ballot papers, out of a total of 333,240, were returned undelivered (approximately 20 per cent) "the main causes of this being the substitution of a consolidated retention fee for an annual retention fee and the failure of nurses to inform the Council of changes of address". Only 64,000 ballot papers were returned—for the first time this figure was less than the number of undelivered ballot papers. 1,271 votes were invalid for various reasons. The election was expected to cost £15,000 and in fact cost £18,280.

Those elected or returned unopposed were:

General seats

Area	Name	Post held
Newcastle	Miss L. B. Stanton	Principal Tutor, Darlington Memorial Hospital
Leeds	Miss G. E. Watts	Matron, The General Infirmary, Leeds
Sheffield	Miss P. Goodall	Principal Tutor Leicester Royal Infirmary
East Anglia	Miss M. J. D. Cooper	Principal Tutor, Addenbrooke's Hospital
N.W. Metropolitan	Miss M. Scott Wright	Matron, Middlesex Hospital

N.E. Metropolitan	Miss P. M. Friend	Matron, The London Hospital
S.E. Metropolitan	Miss B. B. Whyte	Principal Tutor, Guy's Hospital
S.W. Metropolitan	Miss R. A. Hone	Principal Tutor, St. Thomas's Hospital
Oxford	Miss M. E. Coombe	Matron, General Hospital, Northampton
South Western	Miss I. M. May	Principal Tutor, The Taunton and Somerset Hospital, Taunton
Wales	Miss M. A. Gough	Principal Tutor, Cardiff Royal Infirmary
Birmingham	Miss M. M. Pearce	Matron, Birmingham General Hospital
Manchester	Miss L. Jones	County Superintendent of District Nurses, Lancashire
Liverpool	—	—
Wessex	Miss M. R. Jones	Matron, Southampton General Hospital

Four members were re-elected and eleven were new.

Mental nurses

Miss D. V. Williams, Matron, Whittingham Hospital, Preston

Mr. A. N. S. Marshall, Charge Nurse, Forest Hospital, Horsham

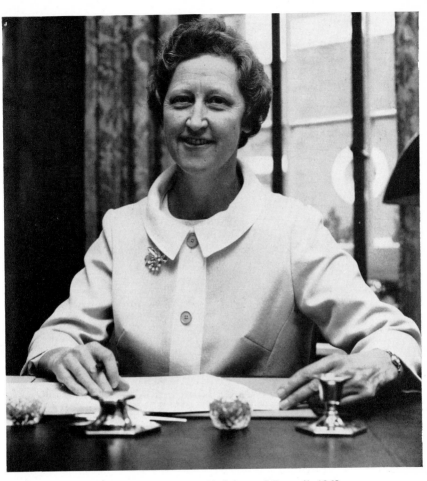

14. Miss Grace Watts, Chairman of Council, 1968.
(By kind permission of the *Nursing Times*).

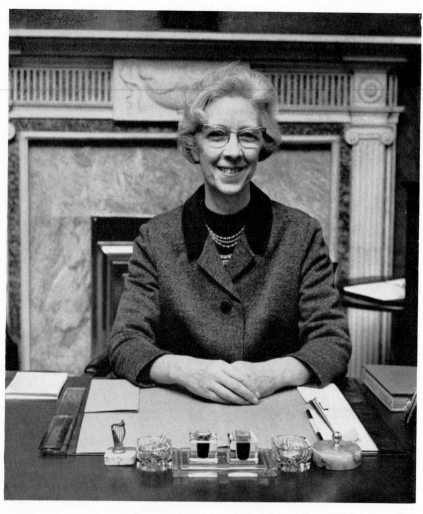

15. Miss Mary Henry, Registrar, 1968.

Sick Children's Nurses

    Miss E. R. D. Bendall, Principal Tutor, The Hospital for Sick Children, Great Ormond Street

All the last three members were new.

One of the first duties of the new Council which met in September 1965 was to appoint a nurse to represent the Liverpool Region, and Miss S. M. Lewis, Matron, Chester Royal Infirmary, accepted the Council's invitation to serve.

The Chairman is Miss G. Watts, and the Vice-Chairman, Miss R. A. Hone.

With reference to the press comment on the numbers of matrons and tutors standing, the numbers elected are as follows:

	Matrons	Tutors
1955	10	2
1960	10	3
1965	8	8

It is fascinating to study the composition of the elected section of the nine General Nursing Councils for England and Wales and to note the way in which certain hospitals continue to take a vital interest in nursing politics. Even the change in 1949 to regional representation did little to alter this. The influence of St. Bartholomew's Hospital both on the early Councils and their staff is impressive; this was a logical development since many of the early protagonists of registration were associated with this hospital. Equally interesting, in view of their early opposition, is the fact that St. Thomas's Hospital has had a representative on the Council for 43 of its 50 years' history.

Other hospitals with more than 25 years' association with the work of the Council through its members are: Birmingham General Hospital and the group of which it was later a part; Guy's Hospital; Manchester Royal Infirmary; Middlesex Hospital; The General Infirmary at Leeds; and The Hospital for Sick Children, Great Ormond Street, London. A similar link with certain hospitals can be noted in the senior members of the staff—particularly University College Hospital and the Middlesex Hospital.

A HISTORY OF THE GENERAL NURSING COUNCIL

THE MINISTER'S VISIT

On July 28th, 1967, the Minister of Health, the Right Hon. Kenneth Robinson, M.P., paid a visit to the Council's offices. This was the first time for nearly 20 years that any Minister had been to 23 Portland Place.

Mr. Robinson spent two hours touring the offices, and met all the heads of departments and those members of the Council's staff with very long service. He afterwards lunched with members of Council and the senior staff, at a nearby hotel.

Chapter 13

TRENDS

"This is not the end. It is not even the beginning of the end.
But it is, perhaps, the end of the beginning."

WINSTON CHURCHILL

The Constitution of the Council

During 1965 the Council set up an *ad hoc* committee to discuss
and assess the powers and work of the statutory committees.
The members of the *ad hoc* committee were the Chairman and
Vice-Chairman of Council, the Chairman of the Mental Nurses
Committee and the Chairman of the Enrolled Nurses Committee. The committee had been set up to study the problems
involved, now that the work of the three training committees
was to some extent being duplicated; for example, reports of
inspections of hospitals where both students and pupils were
being trained had to be presented to and discussed by two committees, and with the opening of the Roll to those employed in
the psychiatric field a similar overlapping occurred.

There were also two disciplinary bodies and if a nurse was
both registered and enrolled she would have to appear before
both.

It became obvious to the committee that the whole question
of the composition of the Council was involved, and as this was
outside their terms of reference the matter was referred back to
the whole Council.

In the meantime the Registration Committee had been collecting information about the composition and methods of
appointment or election of other statutory bodies. They were
concerned at the numbers of candidates and voters at the 1965
election and pointed out that the electorate in 1970 is likely to
exceed 500,000. The Registration Committee recommended to
Council that another ad hoc committee should be set up, with
full powers to consider and advise on the composition of the
Council and its statutory committees. Council approved the
recommendation. The new *ad hoc* committee had the same
composition as before with the addition of the chairman of
the Registration Committee. This committee submitted their
report to Council in July 1966. The introduction to the report

253

stated that the committee had agreed on certain points:

(1) That the constitution of the Council must be such as to enable it to carry out its statutory duties—e.g. training, examinations and disciplinary functions.

(2) That in view of the changed pattern of training, there should be adequate representation on the Council of those involved in the training of pupil nurses and psychiatric nurses; this could mean that the statutory committees would no longer be necessary, and the Mental Nurses Committee would become a standing committee.

(3) Some members felt that consideration should be given to the Council becoming an all-appointed body. The chairman of the Mental Nurses Committee dissented from this view.

The views of the *ad hoc* committee were put before the statutory committees and the Minister of Health informed that preliminary discussions, which could lead to the need for amending legislation, were taking place.

In September 1966 Council received the views of the Mental Nurses and the Enrolled Nurses Committee, and decided to send the tentative proposals to all relevant organisations, asking for their views. The organisations were:

The 15 Area Nurse-Training Committees.

The Royal College of Nursing.

The Association of Hospital Matrons.

The National Association of Chief Male Nurses.

The Society of Registered Male Nurses.

The British Paediatric Nurses Association.

The Nurse Teachers Association.

The Health Visitors Association.

The Association of District Nurses.

The National Association of State Enrolled Nurses.

The Confederation of Health Service Employees.

The National Association of Local Government Officers.

The National Union of General and Municipal Workers.

The National Union of Public Employees.

The Association of Hospital and Welfare Administrators.

Replies were asked for by January 31st, 1967.

The papers circulated to the bodies mentioned, reiterated the points already made and stressed that:

(a) the Council must remain an autonomous body;

(b) it must have a majority of nurses;

(c) the present electoral system should not be discarded unless this step was essential.

The views of the Enrolled Nurses Committee were included; many deprecated the suggestion that the committee should cease to exist, but said that if it did the Council should include two State Enrolled Nurses. They also felt that elections should continue and were supported in this view by members of the Mental Nurses Committee.

The organisations were asked to answer nine specific questions and were finally asked for any further comments.

Full details were published in the nursing journals.

Replies were received from all but one of the organisations and a summary of replies discussed by the *ad hoc* committee; their views were then sent to the statutory committees and finally, at the Council meeting in March 1967, there was discussion of the whole matter, to which those members of the statutory committees who were not members of Council, were invited. Council decided to incorporate those changes suggested by the majority of the profession, as represented by the organisations, and to forward the final suggestions to them and to the Ministry, with a request to the latter for a meeting for further discussion. The Council's annual report for 1966–7 states: "that the possibility of an all-appointed Council is not being proceeded with; with the exception of three Area Nurse-Training Committees, all the bodies consulted were against this proposal."

The proposals forwarded, which were still only regarded as being "in their very preliminary stages" included:

(1) The formation of a mental nurses standing committee in place of the present statutory committee, with provision for adequate representation on the Council of registered mental nurses and nurses of the mentally subnormal. The standing committee to have a majority of psychiatric nurses.

(2) The cessation of the Enrolled Nurses Committee, whose work would be taken over by the Council, and its standing committees, with adequate representation on the Council of registered and enrolled nurses concerned with the training of pupil nurses.

(3) Various ideas to overcome election difficulties, including
the suggestion that those eligible to vote should apply for
ballot papers, rather than these being sent to the whole
electorate.

The constitution of the Council to be:

Appointed members: 18

Department of Education and Science	2
Privy Council	2
Minister of Health	12

to include 3 medical practitioners (1 psychiatric)
2 hospital administrators
4 registered nurses engaged in pupil
nurse training (2 general,
2 psychiatric)
1 district nurse involved in student or
pupil nurse training
2 unspecified

Central Midwives Board	1
Health Visitors Training Council	1

a health visitor or health visitor tutor

Elected members: 22

1 State Registered Nurse from each region elected by S.R.N.s and R.F.N.s	15
1 Registered Sick Children's Nurse to be elected by R.S.C.N.s	1
3 Registered Mental Nurses to be elected by R.M.N.s	3
1 Registered Nurse of the Mentally Subnormal to be elected by R.N.M.S.	1
2 State Enrolled Nurses to be elected by S.E.N.s	2

It was suggested that all doctors and nurses on the Council
should be associated with nurse-training.

It may be of interest to compare the foregoing with other
statutory bodies.

Statutory body	No. of members	Size of electorate	Cost of election (where known)
General Medical Council	47 members 36 appointed 11 elected	58,500	£2,000 (1956)

General Dental Council	26 members 15 appointed 11 elected	16,000	20 per cent less than G.N.C. in proportion to size
Council for professions supplementary to medicine	21 members all appointed	(25,000)	—
General Optical Council	30 members 23 appointed 7 elected	8,500 approx.	£290
Central Midwives Board	16 members all appointed	—	—
Council for training of Health Visitors	28 members all appointed	—	—
General Nursing Council for England and Wales 1965	36 members 18 elected 18 appointed	300,000 approx.	£18,000
Joint Nursing and Midwives Council for N. Ireland	20 members 7 appointed 13 elected	10,657	—

There was remarkably little comment on the proposals in the nursing press except on two points although much space was given to the subject in both the *Nursing Times* and the *Nursing Mirror*. One was the proposal to have an all appointed Council which was resisted; the other the proposals relating to the Mental Nurses Committee—about which questions were asked in the House of Commons. In fact, looking at the new proposals, it would appear that mental nurses would be better represented than ever before.

Finance

During the Council's deliberations on the reconstitution, consideration was given to the possibility of returning to an annual retention fee for the Register and the Roll and this subject has been discussed on subsequent occasions. When the annual retention fee was abandoned in 1949 it was 2s. 6d. per year per nurse, with some 120,000 nurses on the Register and Roll; annual registration cost the Council 4s. 7d. per head. The number of nurses has now risen to some 435,000 (registered and enrolled). Without a considerable amount of research it is impossible to know what the collection of annual retention fees would cost now, but the Scottish General Nursing Council is running at a loss, with an annual fee of 16s., and their total number of nurses is smaller than that for England and Wales in 1949. For the General Nursing Council to return to this method, it would appear that they would require either a large increase in staff, or the installation of a computer system involving a heavy capital outlay, or to make use of some system like the Post Office GIRO.

The Council's financial problems over nurse training came to a head in 1967. The amount of money allowed for salaries of teaching staff has always been estimated on the number of staff in post, plus those expected to complete the appropriate courses. During 1966–7 overspending on salaries occurred to the extent of £26,875. This was due to an unexpected and un-foreseeable increase in the number of established teaching posts filled, which probably resulted from an increase in the number of nurses in training attributable to the Ministry's advertising campaign. Most of the new "teachers" were not qualified as such. When this trend became apparent, and in view of the general financial situation in the country at that time, Council discussed methods of controlling overspending; they reluctantly decided that it was not possible to make an approach to the Ministry for more money at that time and they advised the A.N.T.C.s that for the time being they must restrict the filling of established teaching staff posts to those with teaching qualifications. Unqualified tutors could only be appointed with the approval of the Finance Committee. The Area Nurse-Train-ing Committees were not happy at this restriction but agreed to co-operate.

Even these steps did not prove sufficient and the Council finally had to approach the Ministry for additional money to cover those in post and those who qualified as tutors in August 1967.

During 1967 the Minister indicated that he would be willing

to give a grant for a five-year period to finance the setting up of a small research unit at the General Nursing Council. A steering committee consisting of members of Council, of representatives of the Ministry and of an outside adviser who is an expert in educational research, has been set up, to appoint staff and oversee the programme.

Training

The future pattern of nurse training is debatable and no two nurses will necessarily agree about it. Too many questions remain unanswered and too few statistics are available. From 1860 onwards hospitals have complained that they are short of nursing staff, but what they mean is that they are short of "pairs of hands". No one has ever defined, to everyone's satisfaction, the duties of a trained nurse, the true concept of a student nurse, non-nursing duties, the nurse/patient ratio in different types of units, or how to relate supply to demand. In the 1920s after the passing of the Registration Act, it was hoped that patients could be cared for by a staff of Registered nurses and probationers in training; in the 1940s the hopes lay with the new grade of Enrolled Assistant Nurse. The 1950s brought the term "other nursing staff", and the 1960s have seen even the favoured teaching hospitals advertising for all grades of staff. Almost certainly, there will never be enough to fulfil everyones "needs", and so it would be more realistic to make the best use of what we have.

Earlier in this book, reference was made to the fact that when many hospitals were founded the prime considerations were premises and medical treatment and little thought was given as to who would carry out the individual care of patients. To a certain extent this is true today; new units are planned and built to cope with the increasing development of specialities, with little thought as to who is to care for the patient. Despite the endeavours of the Wood Committee, the Platt Committee and to a large extent the General Nursing Council, the nurse in training is still first an employee and second a trainee; neither in medicine, nor in the professions supplementary to medicine would this position be tolerated. Many attempts to improve the training of the student nurse have met with opposition from doctors and administrators for the sole reason that they fear a reduction in the numbers of available staff and therefore the closure of beds. Those facts which are available (e.g. the report of the Glasgow experimental scheme) prove that when training is considered as a primary object, recruitment is good, wastage and sickness are low and the end product as good if not better.

The profession—and future General Nursing Councils—must decide what they want; a continuation of the pattern of the past 50 years—or a radical change. In the next 15 years the number of young people becoming 18 (or $17\frac{1}{2}$) will fall gradually; the 1965 figures will not be reached again until 1980. These facts have been circulated to hospitals by the Ministry of Health.

Certain specific problems must be solved; the educational level of entry; the age of entry; the length of training; the content of training; the size of training schools; and the type of trained nurse we wish to produce.

The Platt Committee suggested that the educational level of entry to student nurse training should be five O Levels, and it is true that many headmistresses are dismayed by the present minimum of two O Levels and advise their "academic girls" to chose other careers. However, the General Nursing Council are only too well aware of the present position; in 1966 they circulated training schools to ask for details of actual educational requirements for entry to student nurse training. The results were interesting; of 462 training schools, 14 could ask (and obtain students with) five or more O Levels; 19 could ask for four O Levels; 24 could ask for three O Levels and 405 asked for Council's minimum—i.e. two O Levels or a pass in the entrance test. It is thought that the raising of the pass mark in the Council's test in 1968 will affect recruitment in over 300 training schools.

It is hoped that many candidates will choose the two-year training for State Enrolment but this in itself raises problems—since not all the profession have fully accepted the S.E.N. as a trained nurse.

There is no doubt that many young people of A Level standard are attracted to nursing, but unless attempts are made to make training and future prospects sufficiently stimulating they will not stay.

The age of entry is highly controversial and many feel that candidates are lost because of the gap between school and training; however, as a means of attracting greater numbers this seems to have little relevance, since presumably it is the same group who reach 17 one year, and 18 the next. The problems of attracting recruits, and keeping students remain.

From 1880 onwards, most nurse training schools favoured three years as the best training period, and this was incorporated in the Rules following the 1919 Nurses Act. When this period was first introduced, the three years included a 60–70-hour week, a day off once a month, and usually one week's holiday a year and no time in the school except for preliminary training; this meant some 9,000 hours in contact with the patient, during training. Over the years the hours have been reduced and regulated and the student now works a 42-hour week, has 13 weeks holiday during training and spends some 24 weeks in the school. As a result she has some 5,000 hours in contact with the patient.

During the same period, the pattern of nursing and the whole nature of work in the hospital has changed dramatically. In the last 20 years developments in anaesthetics, antibiotics and other drugs, and surgical techniques have reduced both the length of time the patient is kept in bed, and his stay in hospital. Combined with the shorter working week and the change in most off-duty systems, this means that nurses in training rarely take part in the total care of any one patient and as a result their learning and experience are fragmented. When future patterns of nurse training are being considered, these points must be borne in mind.

The content of the syllabus of training must reflect the pattern of disease and social conditions. For the first half of the Council's history, there was little need for radical change since the problems remained much the same and were those connected with infection and communicable disease, hygiene, and the needs of the patient confined to bed. Since the war (1939–45) there have been dramatic changes; the increase in the birth rate, leading to an increased emphasis on obstetrics and neonatal care; the stress disorders and the need for understanding of human behaviour in illness; the rise in the number of old people and the present emphasis on the care and rehabilitation of the elderly; and the rapid development of the use of drugs, and of the specialities. The syllabuses of training for all the Registers were changed between 1957 and 1964 and are already under review again. With the current changes in the grouping of patients, a change in the Council's requirements for practical experience is likely; in the past, it has been easy to label wards male or female, medical or surgical or "speciality"; in the future, the grouping may well be intensive care, intermediate care and minimal care units. Whatever the length of training— two, three or four years—no student or pupil can possibly cover every speciality, and it is useless to give too little practical experience in any unit. Either the training pattern must be far more flexible, or the profession must decide what is necessary in a basic course, and must accept that the newly registered or enrolled nurse is in no way an expert in every field.

Closely connected with the last subject is the proposed future development of the hospital service. In 1962 a hospital plan for England and Wales was published, and although this has since been changed, the tendency is towards the development of district general hospitals with an optimum size of 600–800 beds. Quite apart from the building programme there is a gradual grouping of hospitals to form larger (and fewer) overall units. This will inevitably alter the size and complexity of nurse training schools, and thus bring about closure of some. Although large schools of nursing have many advantages there are problems in grouping hospitals with no thought for nurse training. The Council's policy has always been to advise the formation of a group school only when an individual hospital could not provide adequate practical experience; grouping for other reasons can lead to frequent unnecessary moves for student and pupil nurses with an associated rise in the wastage and sickness rates. The advantages of group schools result from a better distribution of teaching staff, cross-fertilisation of ideas and centralisation of equipment and books.

One of the most important points to be decided in the next few years is the question of reciprocal registration between this and other countries especially the European Economic Community. If Great Britain joins the Common Market, free movement of labour is a sine qua non. As mentioned in an earlier chapter, discussions have been taking place for the last few years, and already the United Kingdom Government has signed the European Agreement. At the present time, the two years training for State Enrolment is not recognised for membership of the International Council of Nurses, let alone the Council of Europe. Although the Council (G.N.C.) is not required to consider the United States of America and Canada (or any other country) when planning training programmes, it is a fact that an increasing proportion of newly registered nurses expect to be able to register abroad in the country of their choice. Contrary to popular opinion, State Registration does not automatically guarantee this, and many who travel to other countries without preliminary investigation, find themselves working as unqualified auxiliaries while they undertake further training and/or examinations.

In this country, at the moment, the main new addition to the syllabus is likely to be principles of management as mentioned in the Salmon Committee Report on senior nursing staff structure (1966). The G.N.C. published its comments on this report early in 1967. In the main the Council were in favour of the proposals in the report, but felt that there was a great need for flexibility; in addition the Council put forward certain points relating to teaching staff whom it was felt should have an entirely separate grading structure.

Examinations

There has been little radical change in the pattern of the Council's examinations for many years, although in the last ten years new methods have been introduced in the general educational field. One of the Council's biggest problems has been that, as one of the largest examining bodies in the country, it is extremely difficult to maintain an even standard. In an endeavour to overcome this, and after a detailed experiment, a new system of marking written papers (grades instead of marks) was introduced in October 1966 and it may be that in the future, objective type (multiple choice) questions will take the place of the present essay, or structured answers.

Even greater difficulties are experienced in regard to the "practical" examination. Quite apart from the enormous problems experienced by the Council's examination department in finding sufficient suitable examiners who are free to examine, busy schools of nursing are faced two or three times a year with their normal teaching responsibilities, plus being an examination centre, plus sending one or more tutors away to examine at other places. The current practical examination is entirely artificial and to overcome this, many examiners use the time available for an oral test based on the candidate's practical experience. Following discussions with the Tutor Section of the Rcn and the Association of Hospital Matrons' the Council have experimented with examinations in hospital wards at selected centres in 1967 and 1968. Everyone concerned with these experiments met for discussion and it is likely that certain changes will result. The use, in a final assessment, of student nurses' ward reports, is a controversial topic.

Summary

It will be obvious to the reader that part of this chapter is factual and the rest is surmise. Any opinions expressed are those of the authors who because of the nature of their work have a special interest in nurse training.

Looking back over the period covered by this book one is struck by two things: first, the tremendous amount achieved by the General Nursing Council against formidable opposition; second, the strengths and weaknesses of a statutory body. Even within the nursing profession, few realise the time taken to collect information and reach agreement before requesting amending legislation—in itself an extremely lengthy business. Once new legislation is achieved its wording is totally binding and not always entirely what was expected.

It is perhaps unfortunate that in its early days the Council provoked enormous publicity and has since shunned it, and even in 1968 there are a great many trained nurses who do not know what the Council does, who its members are, or where its offices are situated.

One of the criticisms of the early Councils was that many of its members had retired from active work. Today this is no longer possible since both elected and appointed nurses must be in post at the time of their election, or appointment. While this is essential, since it ensures that they are in touch with current thought and practice, it means that they are unable to devote as much time as they would like to meeting members of the pro-

16. The Council in session, 1968.

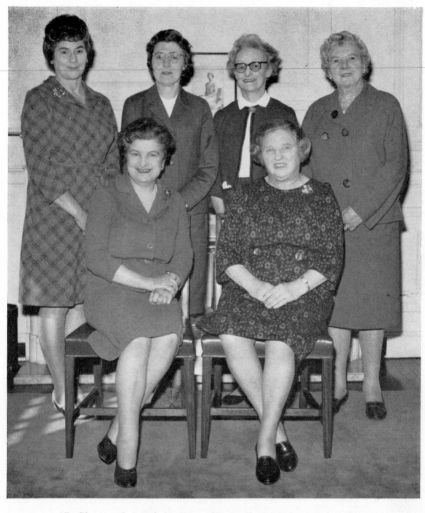

17. Six members of the Council's staff with long service, 1968
(see Appendix 4).

Standing, left to right; Mrs. Hall, Miss Warren, Mrs. Cameron, Mrs. Gorton
Sitting; Miss Ledger, Miss Frazer.

fession. In addition to full-time work, the Chairman and Vice-Chairman of Council attend between 80–100 meetings each year, and those who serve on several committees and sub-committees between 40–60.

In 1969 the General Nursing Council will celebrate its Jubilee. It is to be hoped this will to some extent re-awaken the profession's interest in its statutory body and the subsequent elections in 1970. In many ways the General Nursing Council for England and Wales is unique because of the breadth of its responsibilities and the size of its Register and Roll.

EPILOGUE

Res ipsa loquitor.

When describing the history of any organisation such as the General Nursing Council, it is inevitable that the names and personalities mentioned are those of members of Council and its senior executive officers. It is also inevitable that most of the day-to-day work is carried out by the permanent staff of the office, who are rarely recognised or known.

By the end of 1927, the Council's staff numbered 46; by the mid-1960s this number had risen to over 200. Today the work in the office is divided between various departments; the names given are those of senior officers in post at the beginning of 1968.

REGISTRAR'S OFFICE I

This department is headed by the deputy Registrar, Miss E. Perrin Brown, and is divided into the committee and disciplinary section and the general office. It services the Council and its committees in arranging meetings, preparing agenda, drafting minutes and documents for consideration, handling correspondence after meetings and maintaining and indexing minute books. The staff carry out the necessary research into precedents, official documents and legislation. This department also deals with appointments, correspondence concerning pay, conditions of service and other establishment matters for certain grades of staff, and also maintains records and correspondence relating to retired members of staff whose pensions are paid by the Council.

The staff of this office are responsible for the sealing of documents, the marshalling of material relating to documents to be drafted by the Registrar, all matters relating to disciplinary procedures affecting registered and enrolled nurses, student and pupil-nurses, and persons posing as registered or enrolled nurses.

During 1967, 151 items were on the agenda for consideration by the Investigating Committee; 115 items were on the agenda for consideration by the Disciplinary Committee; and 75 disciplinary items were on the agenda for consideration by the Enrolled Nurses Committee.

During each quinquennial period the office staff deal with all correspondence in connection with the appointment or election of members of Council or its statutory committees.

The general office provides a typing, stencilling, duplicating and photocopying service for the Council, its committees and the Education Department.

REGISTRAR'S OFFICE 2

This department is under the control of the assistant Registrar, Miss E. Johnson, and its work may be summarised under the following headings:

(1) General
(2) Uniform applications
(3) Post room
(4) Reception
(5) Printing.

General

This covers the recruitment and welfare of all staff (clerical and domestic), other than those senior clerical staff who are under the aegis of Registrar's office 1. The number of clerical staff fluctuates between 200 and 240, depending on whether elections, or a major project such as the opening of the Roll to psychiatric nurses are in progress. It also covers the maintenance of the Council's premises, the purchase of furniture, equipment and stationery, and all domestic matters including the supervision of the staff canteen.

The uniform and publications section

(a) Despatches badges to all State Registered and Enrolled nurses; approximately 17,500 S.R.N. badges and 11,500 S.E.N. badges are issued annually.

(b) Deals with all correspondence relating to lost badges and the subsequent issue of duplicate badges: approximately 300 duplicate S.R.N. badges and 100 duplicate S.E.N. badges annually.

(c) Deals with the issue of agreement forms to firms who are authorised by the Council to supply uniform to registered and enrolled nurses.

(d) Maintains records in connection with the above.

(e) Maintains records and stocks of all the Council's publications, e.g. syllabuses and supplements to the Register or Roll.

(f) Prepares and despatches all orders for publications, involving about 275,000 items annually.

The post room staff deal with all incoming and outgoing post:

Incoming post—about 264,000 letters annually

Outgoing post—about 367,500 letters annually.

In addition, elections add to the work of the department as follows:

1963 Enrolled Nurses election—58,479 letters posted

1965 Council members election—333,000 letters posted

1965 Mental Nurses election—33,000 letters posted.

Reception

There are two telephonist/receptionists; they deal with an average of 26,000 incoming telephone calls and 15,600 outgoing telephone calls each year. In addition, they are the first people to receive and direct over 4,000 nurses who call at the Council's offices each year, mostly in connection with registration.

Printing

Apart from confidential examination matters, syllabuses and other booklets sold from the publications department, all letter headings and most of the printed forms in use, are printed on the Council's premises; about 489,000 items are printed annually.

THE REGISTRATION DEPARTMENT

This department is headed by the Registration and Enrolment Officer, Miss E. M. Moore, whose assistants are Miss E. Dodsworth and Miss G. A. Houghton. It is responsible for issuing registration and enrolment numbers, the subsequent issue of certificates and the maintenance of the manuscript Register. The manuscript Register is still handwritten, and two persons are permanently employed on this. For day-to-day use, a Kardex system is kept, in which there is a card for every nurse whose name appears on the Register or Roll of Nurses maintained by the Council.

The work of the department covers the following points:

(a) Change of name due to marriage—about 4,900 annually;

(b) re-inclusion of names to the Register; this applies to those nurses who did not pay the life fee in 1950; these numbers have increased as many nurses, who have married and brought up families, are now returning to active nursing— approximately 280 annually;

(c) change of name by legal document;

(d) issue of duplicate certificates;

(e) application for the Council's certificate of registration as a Teacher of Nurses;

(f) application for initial registration by examination— about 13,200 each year;

(g) application for registration by nurses trained abroad— about 5,000 annually;

(h) maintenance of monthly and annual statistics;

(i) removal of names from the Register because of death;

(j) verification of registration of Nurses Boards overseas— for those nurses going abroad—about 5,450 annually;

(k) preparation and checking of proofs for additions to the Register of Nurses—three times a year;

(l) micro-filming of records; all early records have now been filmed. This work is almost entirely carried out by retired nurses working on a part-time basis.

The work of the enrolled nurses section is similar to that described for the Register, although the numbers involved are smaller. Applications are still received from "existing assistant nurses".

The department handles numerous telephone calls, most of which require confirmation that a nurse is in fact registered or enrolled.

The Registration Officer is in attendance at all meetings of the Registration Committee and its sub-committees.

THE EDUCATION DEPARTMENT

The Education Department is headed by the Education Officer, Miss B. N. Fawkes, and her professional staff are the assistant Education Officer, Miss M. R. Briggs and eight Inspectors of Training Schools. The work of the department is closely linked with that of the three training committees and deals with matters relating to approval of training schools, educational requirements for entry to training, preparation of syllabuses, the type and content of examinations and assessments and the appointments of members of the Boards of Examiners and of the Panel of Examiners and Assessors. The committees and officers are also concerned with transfers or reductions in training for individual student and pupil-nurses, sick and special leave allowed for those in training, approval of courses preparing teachers of nursing, and the content of compulsory refresher courses for tutors and teachers of pupil nurses.

The Education Officers are responsible for advising the committees on all matters under consideration, and help training schools to solve problems relating to training, examinations or assessments. This work necessitates frequent discussion with hospital authorities, which may take place at the training school concerned or in the Council's offices. The officers put forward the Council's policy for training by speaking to varied groups of nurses or others interested in training, e.g. at Area Nurse-Training Committee meetings, conferences or study days; they also serve as members of steering committees preparing experimental schemes of training and as members of advisory committees such as the University of London Extra Mural Advisory Committee on Sister Tutor Diplomas. They lecture to students attending courses in teaching or administration.

One of the Education Officers is in attendance at all meetings of the training committees and their various sub-committees, at meetings of Boards of Examiners and Assessors, and when applicants are being interviewed for the Panel of Examiners or Assessors.

The Inspectors of Training Schools are in attendance at training committee meetings to present their reports on visits of inspection to training schools. The inspectors each work in all areas of England and Wales, but once an inspector has visited a particular hospital or group of hospitals, she/he continues to be responsible for visiting and advising that hospital. Two of the inspectors hold the appropriate qualifications in psychiatric nursing and so devote most of their time to the psychiatric field, and at least one and usually two of the inspectors are Registered Sick Children's Nurses and can advise on this branch of nursing.

THE EXAMINATIONS DEPARTMENT

The Examinations Department is under the control of the Examinations Officer, Miss L. Fleming and two assistant Examinations Officers, Miss M. Gretton and Miss D. Stevens. The work can be described under the following headings:

(1) General
(2) The Index of student and pupil nurses
(3) The examinations for student nurses
(4) The assessments of pupil nurses.

General

The officers arrange accommodation for examinations and call-up of examiners, the planning of timetables, and the dispatch of all notifications to training schools and to examiners. They pack and dispatch the actual question papers, collate the results and compile statistics. In addition to correspondence relating to the work of specific sections of the department, the officers deal with about 90 miscellaneous enquiries per day. They handle all correspondence relating to applications from nurses wishing to be examiners or assessors, make arrangements for interviews, and one officer is in attendance at the interviewing sessions.

The Examinations Officer arranges meetings of Boards of Examiners and Assessors, and is in attendance at the meetings of the examinations sub-committee.

The index of student and pupil nurses

All index forms are received and checked by this section and index numbers are issued. The length and training, whether full or reduced, is verified at this stage and the numbers are notified to the heads of training schools. Notifications of discontinuations are listed monthly, as are statistics of intake and withdrawal. The approximate numbers per annum handled by the section are:

	Intake	Withdrawal	Re-admission
Student nurses	19,500	7,550	1,000
Pupil nurses	9,920	3,240	250

The examinations for student nurses

The dates of the statutory examinations are planned three years in advance. The cycle of work involved for each examination takes four months and must be strictly timed. Three weeks are allowed for application for and return of entry forms; a further three to four weeks for the checking and listing of candidates, followed by the preparation of packs of question papers and materials for each examination centre; arrangements are made for 300 written centres taking some 12,000 candidates, and 120 practical centres taking some 7,500 candidates. Mark sheets are prepared and sent to examiners.

Once the examination has been completed, the results are gradually compiled; all scripts are marked by two examiners and if they fail to agree, the scripts are re-marked by a special committee; this, at present, involves about 1,000 answer books on each occasion. Result letters are sent to individual candidates and heads of training schools about six weeks after the examination takes place.

The assessment of pupil nurses

The dates of the assessments are planned a year in advance and the cycle of events at each assessment is similar to that already described for student nurses. At each assessment, at present, there are some 3,500 entrants and as about 25 per cent are undertaking a reduced period of training between one and six months, all these cases have to be investigated and recorded during the preparation for the assessment.

As the assessment does not take place at the end of the two-year period of training, much work has to be repeated when the pupil nurse applies for enrolment.

The section receives about 100 letters a week regarding training and transfer.

THE FINANCE DEPARTMENT

The financial administrator is Mr. J. C. Davis, and the accountant Miss C. A. Raybould; both these officers attend meetings of the Finance Committee and its sub-committees. The work of the department can be described under the following headings:

(1) Collecting income
(2) Settlement of liabilities
(3) Nurse-training funds
(4) Investments.

Income

The Council's income is derived mainly from fees for examinations, assessments, registration and enrolment. This involves a yearly total of some £400,000, made up of some 150,000 remittances, most of which arrive at the offices during only 12 weeks of the year. The remaining income comes from the sale of publications, investment income, rents from property let and payments made by the Minister of Health for approval and inspection of training schools. Fees are also received from the disclaimed hospitals.

Liabilities

The largest portion of the Council's liabilities is staff salaries and wages. Payment of fees and expenses to examiners and assessors is a major exercise for the department since, like the income, activity is spasmodic, involving three short spells of extreme pressure.

Nurse-training funds

The mechanics of accounting for nurse-training funds (received yearly from the Ministry of Health), is a relatively straightforward exercise, but providing the data for its control is more difficult. Much statistical information is obtained, collated and kept up to date for a continuous appraisal of the probable end-of-year result, so that appropriate action can be taken to attempt to keep expenditure in line with funds allocated.

Investments

The Council's investments are discussed at a sub-committee attended by the financial experts on the Finance Committee and members of Council, who are advised by the Council's broker. The introduction of the Capital Gains Tax has made the need for accurate records much more important, so that losses may be realised to offset gains.

It is interesting to note that the Council is an earner of foreign exchange and "trained abroad" applications involve transactions in currencies throughout the non-communist world.

Date	Council's annual income	Value of net assets
	£	£
31.3.21	169	—
31.3.22	5,809	—
31.3.23	23,162	—
31.3.24	31,608	—
31.3.25	27,505	34,018
31.3.30	38,349	70,735
31.3.35	47,673	110,855
31.3.40	43,045	168,236
31.3.45	104,603	160,011
31.3.50	149,505	126,774
31.3.55	143,379	739,427
31.3.60	211,061	918,525
31.3.65	231,625	871,720
31.3.66	328,097	834,935
31.3.67	432,128	866,946

CONCLUSION

Although the work of the Council's staff has of necessity been described under departmental headings, the work of the whole office, under the leadership and management of its Registrar, Miss Mary Henry, is closely linked.

A student or pupil-nurse is first indexed with the examinations department; she follows a prescribed syllabus and her training school is inspected by members of the education department. At some point she/he will enter for one of the Council's examinations and her fee will be received and recorded by the finance department. On the successful completion of training, the registration department will handle her application for registration or enrolment, and on payment of her fee she will receive the Council's publication on disciplinary procedure, and her badge, certificate and uniform permit. Should she wish to work abroad, her registration will be confirmed.

As the years pass, she may obtain a further statutory

qualification, may apply to be an examiner or assessor, may be appointed to the Board of Examiners, or be appointed or elected a member of Council, or become one of its officers.

On the fourth Friday of January, March, May, July, September and November, at 2.30 p.m. any members of the nursing profession or general public can go to 23 Portland Place, London, W.1, and take their place in the public gallery of the Council chamber, to listen to the proceedings of the formal meeting of the General Nursing Council for England and Wales. The meeting rarely takes more than one hour, but it is the culmination of tremendous activity in committee and in the Council's offices over the preceding two months.

Appendix 1(i)

MEMBERS OF COUNCIL 1920–1968

(E—elected, A—appointed. *—Still a member of the Council)

Alsop	Miss H. A.	S.R.N.	1923–1932	E
Armstrong	Miss K.	S.R.N.	1926–1927	A
Alexander	Miss C. H. now Lady Mann	O.B.E.; S.R.N.	1945–1950	E
Allison	Miss K. M.	S.R.N.	1960–1965	E
Bostock Hill	Dr. A.	M.D.	1920–1922	A
Barratt	Miss A. S.		1923–1925	A
Bremner	Miss G.	S.R.N.	1923–1932	E
Bushby	Miss A. M.	R.S.C.N.; S.R.N.	1923–1932	E
Barratt	Lady	C.B.E., M.D.	1928	A
Blackman	Mr. E. R.	R.M.N.	1928–1932	E
Brown	Miss J.	R.M.N.	1928–1932	E
Buchan	Dr. J. J.	M.D.; D.P.H.	1928–1931	A
Bowling	Miss W.	S.R.N.	1933–1937	E
Buckley	Mr. J. H.	J.P.; R.M.N.	1933–1950	E
Bowes	Miss G. M. see Mrs. Whitehurst	S.R.N.	1938–1939	E
Burgess	Miss A.	M.B.E.; A.R.R.C.; S.R.N.	1938–1944	E
Brain	Sir W. Russell	D.M.; F.R.C.P.	1943–1947	A
Barnes	Mr. S. W.		1947–1950	A
Bomford	Dr. R. R.	B.A.; D.M.; F.R.C.P.	1949–1950	A
Baldock	Miss D.	S.R.N.	1950–1954	E
Bartlett	Mr. C.	C.B.E.; R.M.N.	1950–1960	E
Bell	Miss C. F. S.	S.R.N.	1950–1955	E
Bovill	Miss S. C.	S.R.N.	1955–1960	E
Bryant	Miss E. M.	S.R.N.	1955–1958	E
Bell	Miss E. A.		1958–1959	A
Berry	Miss D. J.	S.R.N.	1958–1961	A
Bompas	Mr. R. M.	M.B.E.; A.C.I.S.; F.H.A.	1963*	A
Bendall	Miss E. R. D.	S.R.N.; R.S.C.N.; R.N.T.	1965*	E
Cattell	Miss A.	S.R.N.	1920–1922	A
Christian	Mr. T.	M.P.A.	1920–1922	A
Coulton	Miss A.	S.R.N.	1920–1922	A
Cox-Davies	Miss R. A.	C.B.E.; R.R.C.; S.R.N.	1920–1944	E
Cronshaw	Rev. G. B.	M.A.	1920–1928	A

Coode	Miss D. S.	S.R.N.	1923–1924	E
Cowlin	Miss G.	S.R.N.	1923–1932	E
Collins	Dr. M. A.	C.B.E.; M.D.	1932–1942	A
Cockeram	Miss E.	A.R.R.C.; R.S.C.N.; S.R.N.	1933–1937	E
Courtauld	Mrs. J. S.		1933–1937	A
Campbell	Miss F. M.	R.F.N.; S.R.N.	1939–1948	E
Catnach	Miss A.	C.B.E.; B.A.	1943–1958	A
Calder	Miss J. M. now Mrs. Dossetor	M.B.E.; S.R.N.	1945–1953	E
Craddock	Mr. F. A. W.	M.B.E.; S.R.N. ; R.M.N.	1945–1955	E
Constable	Mr. P. H.	O.B.E.; M.A.; F.H.A.	1950–1962	A
Campbell	Mr. W. G.	B.A.; F.C.A.	1953–1958	A
Cawood	Miss K. I.	O.B.E.; S.R.N.; R.S.C.N.	1955–1965	E
Clark	Miss J. E.	S.R.N.	1960–1965	E
Chambers	Mrs. V. B.	PhD.; J.P.	1961*	A
Coombe	Miss M. E.	S.R.N.	1965*	E
Cooper	Miss M. J. D.	S.R.N.; R.N.T.	1965*	E
Dowbiggin	Miss A.	C.B.E.; R.R.C.; S.R.N.	1920–1922	A
Donaldson	Mr. R.	R.M.N.	1923–1927	E
Du Sautoy	Miss C. C.	S.R.N.	1923–1927	E
Darbyshire	Miss R. E.	R.R.C.; S.R.N.	1933–1937	E
Dey	Miss H.	C.B.E.; R.R.C.; S.R.N.	1933–1950	E
Diamond	Mr. J.	P.C.; F.C.A.; M.P.	1948–1953	A
Darroch	Miss R. B. McK.	M.B.E.; S.R.N.	1950–1958	A
Dixon	Miss N. M.	S.R.N.	1950–1955	E
Daley	Sir A.	B.Sc.; M.B.; Ch.B.; D.P.H.; M.D.; F.R.C.P.	1953–1958	A
Delve	Miss L. E.	S.R.N.; R.M.N.	1953–1965	A
Douglas	Dr. J.	O.B.E.; M.D.; D.P.H.	1958–1966	A
De la Court	Miss L.	M.B.E.; S.R.N.; R.S.C.N.	1962–1965	A
Eason	Sir H.	C.B.; C.M.G.; M.D.; M.S.; F.R.C.S.	1933–1937	A
Erleigh	The Viscountess (later the Marchioness of Reading)		1933–1937	A
Edwards	Hon. Mrs. M. E.		1938–1942	A

Evans	Sir G. A.	M.A.; M.D.; F.R.C.S.	1938–1942	A
Ewing	Dr. J.	M.A.; D.Sc.	1950–1956	A
Evans	Mrs. E.	B.Sc.	1958*	A
Fenwick	Mrs. E. G.	S.R.N.	1920–1922	A
Fawcett	Dr. J.	M.D.; F.R.C.P.; F.R.C.S.	1928–1932	A
Fish	Miss M. E.		1948–1950	A
Forbes	Mrs. M. R.		1948–1950	A
Fulton	Mr. J. S.	M.A.	1955–1959	A
Furze	Miss R. M.	S.R.N.	1960–1965	E
Forest Smith	Dr. J.	F.R.C.P.	1961–1963	A
Friend	Miss P. M.	S.R.N.; R.N.T.	1965*	E
Fairbank	Mr. J.	S.R.N.; R.M.N.; R.N.T.	1965*	A
Goodall	Dr. E. W.	O.B.E.; M.D.	1920–1927	A
Galway	Lady	C.B.E.	1928	A
Gullan	Miss M. A.	S.R.N.	1928–1937	E
Gwatkin	Miss E. R.	M.A.	1933–1942	A
Gooch	Sir H. C.	B.A.; LLB.; J.P.	1938–1947	A
Grant	Miss L. G. Duff	R.R.C.; S.R.N.	1938–1955	E
Graham	Miss A. A.	C.B.E.; S.R.N.	1950–1955	E
Grosvenor	Mr. V. W.	C.B.E.; LLB.; J.P.	1950–1958	A
Graham-Bryce	Dame Isobel	D.B.E.; M.A.; J.P.	1956–1961	A
Goodall	Miss P.	S.R.N.; R.N.T.	1960*	E
Gough	Miss M. A.	S.R.N.; R.N.T.	1960*	E
Gough	Mr. A. Staveley	F.R.C.S.	1963*	A
Herringham	Sir W. P.	K.C.M.G.; C.B.; M.D.; F.R.C.P.	1922–1927	A
Hills	Hon. Mrs. E.		1920–1925	A
Hobhouse	Lady C.		1920–1927	A
Haldane	Miss E. S.	C.H.; LL.D.; J.P.	1928–1932	A
Hogg	Miss M.	C.B.E.; S.R.N.	1928–1932	E
Harper	Mr. W. H.		1933–1937	A
Hillyers	Miss G. V. L.	O.B.E.; S.R.N.	1945–1948	E
Holland	Miss D. L.	S.R.N.	1945–1953 1955–1960	E
Houghton	Miss M.	O.B.E.; S.R.N.	1945–1948	E
Hedges	Miss E. M. now Mrs. Mearns		1950–1958	A
Hume	Mr. J. B.	M.S.; F.R.C.S.	1958–1961	A
Hutchins	Ald. E. C.		1958–1963	A
Hone	Miss R. A.	S.R.N.; R.N.T.	1960*	E
Innes	Miss E. S.	R.R.C.; D.N.; S.R.N.	1933–1937	E

Jones	Miss M.	O.B.E.; A.R.R.C.; M.A.; S.R.N.	1933–1944	E
Jones	Miss L.	M.B.E.; S.R.N.	1955*	E
Jones	Sir Brynmor	Ph.D.; Sc.D.	1961–1966	A
John	Mrs. V. M.	S.R.N.	1963–1966	A
Jones	Mr. Emlyn	M.Sc.; F.R.I.C.	1963*	A
Jones	Miss M. R.	S.R.N.	1965*	E
Kettle	Dr. M. H.	M.R.C.S.; L.R.C.P.	1933–1939	A
Knox	Miss M. M.	S.R.N.	1950–1955	E
Ker	Mr. D. C. A.	B.Comm.; B.Sc.	1953–1963	A
Kirby	Miss G. M.	S.R.N.; R.S.C.N.	1955–1965	E
Knowles	Mrs. E. C.	R.M.N.; R.N.M.D.	1960–1961	E
King	Miss V. M.	S.R.N.	1963*	A
Lloyd Still	Dame Alicia	D.B.E.; R.R.C.; S.R.N.	1920–1937	E
Lord	Lt.-Col. J. R.	C.B.E.; M.D.; F.R.C.S.	1931	A
Limerick	The Countess of	G.B.E.	1933–1950	A
Lane	Miss D. A.	S.R.N.; R.S.C.N.	1938–1955	E
Lawson	Miss M. G.	O.B.E.; M.A.; M.B.; Ch.B.; S.R.N.	1950–1958	A
Lillywhite	Miss F. E.	S.R.N.	1950–1958	A
Loveridge	Miss J. M.	O.B.E.; S.R.N.	1951–1965	E
Lawlor	Mr. F. S.	S.R.N.; R.N.T.	1959*	A
Lewis	Miss S. M.	S.R.N.	1965*	A
MacCallum	Miss M. E.	S.R.N.	1920–1922	A
Macdonald	Miss I.	S.R.N.	1920–1922	A
Musson	Dame Ellen M.	D.B.E.; R.R.C.; LL.D.; S.R.N.	1923–1944	E
Meadows	Miss E. now Mrs. Oakley	S.R.N.	1928–1932	E
Murrell	Dr. C.		1929–1932	A
MacManus	Miss E. E. P.	C.B.E.; S.R.N.	1933–1948	E
Menzies	Sir Frederick	K.B.E.; M.D.; LL.D.; F.R.C.S.; F.R.S.E.	1938–1942	A
Milne	Miss M. E. G.	S.R.N.	1938–1944	E
Macaulay	Dr. H. M. C.	C.B.E.; B.Sc.; M.D.; D.P.H.	1943–1950	A
Monagham	Miss M. A.		1949–1950	A
Marriott	Miss M. J.	O.B.E.; S.R.N.	1950–1965	E
Marshall	Miss W. K.	S.R.N.	1954–1955	A
Morris	Sir Philip	C.B.E.; M.A.; LL.D.	1954–1955	A
Morris	Miss I. H.	S.R.N.	1958–1963	A
Moore	Miss S.	S.R.N.	1958–1963	A

Martin	Sir Albert	C.B.E.	1963*	A
May	Miss I. M.	S.R.N.; R.N.T.	1965*	E
Marshall	Mr. A. N. S.	R.N.M.S.	1965*	E
Montacute	Mr. C.	LL.B.; D.P.A.; F.I.M.T.A.; F.H.A.	1965*	A
Notman	Miss A. G.	S.R.N.; R.S.C.N.; R.N.T.	1963*	A
Noble	Mr. P. S.	M.A.	1961	A
Ousby	Mr. R. J.	S.R.N.	1938–1944	E
Ottley	Miss L. J.	S.R.N.	1950–1960	E
Peterkin	Miss A. M.	C.B.E.; S.R.N.	1920–1922	A
Pierce	Dr. Bedford	M.D.; F.R.C.P.	1920–1927	A
Priestley	Sir Joseph	K.C.	1920–1921	A
Price	Miss M. E.		1926–1927	A
Porter	Dr. C.	M.D.; C.M.; B.Sc.	1932–1937	A
Pearce	Miss E. C.	S.R.N.; R.M.N.	1938–1950	E
Puxley	Miss Z. L.	O.B.E.	1938–1942	A
Picken	Prof. R. M.	M.B.; Ch.B.; D.P.H.	1942–1945 1950–1953	A A
Penson	Prof. Dame Lilian	D.B.E.; Ph.D.	1950–1951	A
Powell	Miss E. M.	S.R.N.	1955–1960	E
Price	Miss J. B.	M.B.E.; S.R.N.; R.N.T.	1955–1960	E
Preddy	Miss E.	S.R.N.	1960–1965	E
Pearce	Miss M. M.	S.R.N.	1965*	E
Powell Phillips	Dr. W.	O.B.E.; M.R.C.S.; L.R.C.P.; D.P.H.	1967*	A
Rees Thomas	Dr. W.	C.B.; M.D.; F.R.C.P.; D.P.M.	1943–1950	A
Rose	Miss A. M.		1944	A
Raven	Dame Kathleen	D.B.E.; S.R.N.	1950–1957	E
Robinson	Miss E.	O.B.E.; S.R.N.	1958*	E
Reynolds	Mrs. P. E.	M.B.E.; S.E.N.	1962*	A
Redman	Miss P.	S.R.N.	1968*	A
Smith	Miss E.	S.R.N.	1920–1927	E
Sparshott	Miss M. E.	C.B.E.; R.R.C.; S.R.N.	1920–1937	E
Swiss	Miss E. C.	S.R.N.	1920–1922	A
Steele	Miss A. T.	M.A.	1921–1922	A
Smedley	Dr. R. D.	M.A.; M.D.	1922–1927	A
Stratton	Mr. F.	S.R.N.	1923–1932	E

Southwell	Mr. J. E.	S.R.N.	1933–1937	E
Smith	Miss D. M.	C.B.E.; S.R.N.	1938–1955	E
Smyth	Miss M. J.	C.B.E.; S.R.N.	1948–1960	E
Sayer	Mr. A. J.	M.B.E.; S.R.N.	1949–1959	A
Sands	Dr. D. E.	M.R.C.P.; L.R.C.S.; D.P.M.	1950–1953	A
Smaldon	Miss C. A.	C.B.E.; S.R.N.	1950–1965	E
Sanderson	Miss A. Y.	S.R.N.	1955–1960	E
Squibbs	Miss A. E. A.	S.R.N.	1957–1960	A
Shaw	Miss F.	O.B.E.; S.R.N.	1960–1965	E
Soley	Mr. J. E.	R.M.N.	1960–1965	E
Stanton	Miss L. B.	S.R.N.; R.N.T.	1965*	E
Tuke	Miss M. J.	M.A.	1920–1921	A
Thomson	Dr. F. H.	M.B.; D.P.H.	1928–1932	A
Tait	Mr. L.	B.A.	1950–1953	A
Todd	Miss J.	M.B.E.; S.R.N.	1950–1955	E
Trayer	Dr. H. G.	M.B.; Ch.B.; D.P.H.	1950–1958	A
Trillwood	Miss E. K.	S.R.N.	1953–1958	A
Tennant	Miss F. I.	S.R.N.	1958–1963	A
Taylor	Dr. A. B.	M.D.; F.R.C.P.	1967*	A
Verrall	Sir T. Jenner	M.R.C.S.; L.R.C.P.	1920–1927	A
Villiers	Miss S. A.	S.R.N.; R.F.N.	1920–1937	E
Worsley	Miss C.	S.R.N.	1920–1922	A
Wiese	Miss M. E.	R.M.N.	1923–1927	E
Wilson	Miss E.		1928–1932	A
Worth	Dr. R.	C.B.E.; M.B.	1928–1930	A
Willis	Miss K. M.	R.M.N.	1933–1950	E
Whitehurst	Mrs. G. M. see Miss Bowes	A.R.R.C.; S.R.N.	1940–1943	E
Walton	Mr. H. M.	M.A.	1943–1947	A
Watt	Dame Katherine	D.B.E.; R.R.C.; S.R.N.	1943–1950	A
Waters	Miss W. V.	S.R.N.; R.N.M.D.	1950–1957	E
Whillis	Prof. J.	M.D.; M.S.; F.R.C.S.	1952–1955	A
Walk	Dr. A.	M.D.; D.P.M.	1953*	A
Williams	Miss D.	S.R.N.	1958–1960	A
Whitbread	Major S.		1958–1965	A
Wilson	Mr. C. H.	M.A.	1959–1961	A
Williams	Miss D. V.	S.R.N.; R.M.N.	1959*	E & A
Watts	Miss G. E.	S.R.N.; R.N.T.	1960*	E
White	Miss D. M.	O.B.E.; S.R.N.	1961*	A

Whyte	Miss B. B.	S.R.N.; R.N.T.	1965–1968	E
Wright	Miss M. Scott	Ph.D.; M.A.; S.R.N.	1965*	E
Walker	Miss M. D.	S.R.N.	1967*	A
Yapp	Miss C. Seymour	S.R.N.	1920–1925	E

The authors have endeavoured to ensure that the information in this list is accurate; if any mistakes have been made this is sincerely regretted.

August 1968,

Appendix 1(ii)

APPOINTED MEMBERS OF STATUTORY COMMITTEES WHO ARE NOT MEMBERS OF COUNCIL

Appointed by the Minister of Health

FINANCE COMMITTEE

Hayhurst	Mr. W.	F.I.M.T.A.; R.S.A.A.	1950*
Todd	Mr. E. D. B.	F.I.M.T.A.; F.C.A.	1965*
West	Mr. A. L. A.	F.I.M.T.A.; A.H.A.	1950–1965

MENTAL NURSES COMMITTEE

Ackner	Dr. B.	M.A.; M.D.; M.R.C.P.; D.P.M.	1960–1966
Barry	Mr. N.	S.R.N.; R.M.N.	1960*
Baggott	Miss E.	S.R.N.; R.M.N.; R.N.T.	1965–1966
Craddock	Mr. F. A. W.	M.B.E.; S.R.N.; R.M.N.	1950–1955
Delve	Miss L. E.	S.R.N.; R.M.N.	1950–1955
Fairbank	Mr. J.	S.R.N.; R.M.N.; R.N.T.	1965
Freudenberg	Dr. R. K.	M.D.; L.R.C.P.; L.R.C.S.; D.P.M.	1967*
Gourdie	Miss M. D.	S.R.N.; R.M.N.	1950–1955
Jones	Mr. W. G.	S.R.N.; R.M.N.	1955–1964
Michell	Miss B. A. C.	S.R.N.; R.M.N.	1955–1965
Melody	Miss B. M.	S.R.N.; R.M.N.	1965*
Rees	Dr. T. P.	O.B.E.; M.D.; M.R.C.P.; D.P.M.	1950–1960
Rogers	Mr. E. J.	S.R.N.; R.M.N.	1955–1960
Sutcliffe	Mr. H.	S.R.N.; R.M.N.; R.N.T.	1967*

ENROLLED NURSES COMMITTEE
(previously the Assistant Nurses Committee)

Brooke	Mrs. B.M.	S.R.N.	1943–1948
Benton	Mr. J. D.	S.E.N.	1950–1953
Butcher	Miss M. G.	S.E.N.	1953–1958
Dreyer	Miss R.	S.R.N.	1943–1948
Ford	Mrs. W. L.	S.R.N.	1943–1948
North	Miss A. D.	S.E.N.	1958–1963
Ramsay	Mr. R. W.	M.B.E.	1948–1953
Reynolds	Mrs. P. E.	M.B.E.; S.E.N.	1960–1963
Snowden	Miss L.	S.R.N.	1943–1948
Tracey	Miss E.	S.E.A.N.	1943–1948
Tucker	Miss M. G.	S.R.N.	1966*
Vosper	Miss A.	R.M.N.; S.E.N.	1948–1950
Wain	Miss O. M.	S.R.N.	1963–1966

* Still a member.

CHAIRMAN AND VICE-CHAIRMAN OF COUNCIL, 1920–1968

Year	Chairman	Vice-Chairman
1920	Mr. J. Priestley, K.C.	—
1921	,,	—
1922	Sir Wilmot Herringham, K.C.M.G.; C.B.; M.D.; F.R.C.P.	—
1923	,,	—
1924	,,	—
1925	,,	—
1926	Miss E. M. Musson, S.R.N.	Sir Wilmot Herringham
1927	,,	,,
1928	,,	Miss R. A. Cox-Davies, S.R.N.
1929	,,	,,
1930	,,	,,
1931	,,	,,
1932	,,	Miss M. E. Sparshott, S.R.N.
1933	,,	Miss R. A. Cox-Davies
1934	,,	,,
1935	,,	Miss R. Darbyshire, S.R.N.
1936	,,	,,
1937	,,	,,
1938	,,	Miss R. A. Cox-Davies
1939	Dame Ellen Musson	Miss D. M. Smith, S.R.N.
1940	,,	,,
1941	,,	,,
1942	,,	,,
1943	,,	,,
1944	Miss D. M. Smith	Dame Ellen Musson
1945	,,	Miss M. Jones
1946	,,	,,
1947	,,	,,
1948	,,	Miss C. H. Alexander, S.R.N.
1949	,,	,,
1950	,,	,,
1951	,,	Miss M. J. Smyth, S.R.N.
1952	,,	,,
1953	,,	,,
1954	,,	,,
1955	Miss M. J. Smyth	Miss J. M. Loveridge, S.R.N.
1956	,,	,,
1957	,,	,,
1958	,,	,,

1959	Miss M. J. Smyth	Miss J. M. Loveridge, S.R.N.
1960	Miss C. A. Smaldon, S.R.N.	,,
1961	,,	,,
1962	,,	Miss R. A. Hone, S.R.N.; R.N.T.
1963	,,	,,
1964	,,	,,
1965	Miss G. E. Watts, S.R.N.	,,
1966	,,	,,
1967	,,	,,
1968	,,	,,

Appendix 3(i)

THE STATUTORY COMMITTEES (August 1968)

The Mental Nurses Committee has 12 members:

> 6 are members of Council
> 2 are Registered Mental Nurses or Registered Nurses of the Mentally Sub-normal, elected by nurses on those parts of the Register
> 4 are appointed by the Minister of Health—3 nurses and 1 doctor

This Committee deals with "any matter which wholly or mainly concerns registered mental nurses (other than a question whether a person shall be registered or shall be removed from or restored to the Register) and any matter relating to the training of persons for admission to that part of the Register."

There is a sub-committee which considers policy with regard to the training of psychiatric nurses.

There are also two joint sub-committees of the Mental Nurses Committee and the Enrolled Nurses Committee.

Members:

Mr. Barry	Mr. O'Leary
Mr. Croney	*Mrs. Reynolds
*Mr. Fairbank	Mr. Sutcliffe
Dr. Freudenberg	*Dr. Walk
*Mr. Marshall (*Chairman*)	*Miss Watts
Miss Melody	*Miss Williams

The Enrolled Nurses Committee has 11 members:

> 6 are members of Council—one at least must not be a registered nurse
> 4 are registered or enrolled nurses elected by enrolled nurses
> 1 is appointed by the Minister

The functions of this Committee are "any matter which wholly or mainly concerns enrolled nurses".

There is a sub-committee to deal with matters regarding training and assessment which also interviews prospective assessors.

Members:

*Miss Coombe	Mr. Snow
Mr. Edwards	Miss Tucker
*Miss Gough (*Chairman*)	*Dr. Walk
Mr. Lane	*Miss Watts
*Mrs. Reynolds	*Miss White
Miss Smith	

* Member of Council.

The Finance Committee has 12 members:

10 are members of Council
2 are nominated by the Minister as being experts in questions of finance

The committee's function is to deal with all financial matters of the Council and the Area Nurse Training Committees.

It has two sub-committees; one deals with the Council's investments and the other with nurse training expenditure.

Members:

*Miss Watts ⎫ *ex-officio* *Miss Hone ⎭	Mr. Hayhurst
	*Mr. Marshall
*Miss Bendall	*Mr. Montacute
*Mr. Bompas (*Chairman*)	*Miss Pearce
*Mrs. Evans	*Miss Robinson
*Miss Friend	Mr. Todd

* Member of Council.

Appendix 3(ii)

THE STANDING COMMITTEES (August 1968)

The Registration Committee has 10 members:

All are members of Council.

The Committee deals, as its name suggests, with all matters concerning registration and has one sub-committee which considers applications from nurses trained abroad.

Members:

Miss Watts ⎱ *ex-officio*	Miss May
Miss Hone ⎰	Miss Notman
Miss Coombe	Miss Pearce
Miss Friend	Miss Robinson (*Chairman*)
Miss M. R. Jones	Miss Williams

The Education and Examinations Committee has 19 members:

All are members of Council.

The Committee is concerned with all matters relating to student nurse training and examinations.

There are three sub-committees; one receives the reports submitted by the Council's inspectors on their visits to the training schools and for the last few years has discussed the various plans submitted for permission to train students under the 1962 syllabus. A second sub-committee on examinations also discusses requests for transfer of training which do not conform to the Council's rules; it appoints Boards of Examiners to set the examination papers and receives all correspondence relating to examinations. The third sub-committee considers experimental schemes of training.

Members:

Miss Watts ⎱ *ex-officio*	Mr. Emlyn Jones
Miss Hone ⎰	Miss M. R. Jones
Miss Bendall (*Chairman*)	Miss Notman
Miss Coombe	Miss Pearce
Miss Cooper	Miss Robinson
Mrs. Evans	Miss Stanton
Miss Friend	Miss White
Miss Goodall	Miss Whyte
Miss Gough	Miss Scott Wright
Mr. Staveley Gough	

288

The Investigating Committee and the Disciplinary Committee work together. The Nurses Rules Approval Instrument 1961 states that: the Investigating Committee shall consist of the Vice-Chairman of Council and five other members none of whom can be members of the Disciplinary Committee.

The Committee reviews all reports of matters concerning registered nurses which could lead to disciplinary action. It advises whether the case shall be heard by the Disciplinary Committee or whether no further action shall be taken.

Members:

Investigating Committee

Mrs. Chambers (*Chairman*)	Mr. Marshall
Mrs. Evans	Dr. Powell Phillips
Miss Hone	Miss Whyte

The Disciplinary Committee consists of the Chairman of Council and 11 other members, two of whom must not be registered nurses. Its Chairman is Chairman of Council.

The Committee deals with all matters referred to it by the Investigating Committee.

Members:

Disciplinary Committee

Mr. Bompas	Sir Albert Martin
Miss Friend	Miss May
Miss L. Jones	Mr. Montacute
Miss King	Dr. Walk
Mr. Lawlor	Miss Watts (*Chairman*)
Miss Lewis	Miss Scott Wright

Appendix 4

Past members of staff with long service to the Council

Name	Last appointment	Years of service
Miss G. E. Davies	Registrar	25½ years
Miss E. M. Falconer	Accountant	28½ years
Miss D. S. Leedham	,,	25½ years
Miss M. O. Bagi	Higher Clerical	35¼ years
Miss D. C. Oakley	,, ,,	38 years
Miss H. Sime	,, ,,	43⅔ years
Miss G. Upton (deceased)	,, ,,	40 years
Miss N. Youngman	Principal Clerk	28½ years
Miss E. Lipscombe	Shorthand Typist	35½ years

Present members of staff with long service to the Council.

Name	Present appointment	Years of service to date
Miss M. G. N. Henry	Registrar	25 years
Miss G. A. Houghton	Assistant Registration Officer	36 years
Miss C. M. Frazer	Higher Clerical	24 years
Mrs. F. E. Gorton	,, ,,	43 years
Miss N. E. Ledger	,, ,,	38 years
Miss I. Warren	,, ,,	31 years
Miss B. Lewis	Clerical Grade	25 years
Miss A. W. Cameron	Higher Clerical (now part-time)	26 years
Mrs. J. Hall	Higher Clerical (some part-time)	24 years

August 1968

INDEX OF STUDENT NURSES IN TRAINING
FOR ALL PARTS OF THE REGISTER

Numbers admitted for the first time each year

At November 30th, 1949	48,469 (from June 1st, 1947)
At March 31st, 1951	27,982 (from November 30th, 1949)
1951–1952	18,734
1952–1953	17,022
1953–1954	17,776
1954–1955	18,920
1955–1956	18,984
1956–1957	20,265
1957–1958	19,808
1958–1959	19,925
1959–1960	19,783
1960–1961	18,992
1961–1962	19,810
1962–1963	20,560
1963–1964	18,260
1964–1965	19,551
1965–1966	19,914
1966–1967	19,547
1967–1968	18,366

Appendix 5(ii)

INDEX OF PUPIL NURSES

Numbers admitted for the first time each year.

February 1946–November 30th, 1949	3,027
November 30th, 1949–March 31st, 1951	2,200
1951–1952	2,119
1952–1953	2,497
1953–1954	2,534
1954–1955	2,729
1955–1956	2,655
1956–1957	3,047
1957–1958	3,165
1958–1959	3,847
1959–1960	4,043
1960–1961	4,054
1961–1962	4,292
1962–1963	5,621
1963–1964	5,584
1964–1965	6,771
1965–1966	8,449
1966–1967	10,229
1967–1968	11,437

N.B.—In 1966 the Index of Pupil Nurses included, for the first time, pupils training in mental and mental sub-normality hospitals.

Appendix 5(iii)

DISCONTINUATION FROM TRAINING AMONG STUDENT AND PUPIL NURSES

	Students entered	Students discontinued	Per cent	Pupils entered	Pupils discontinued	Per cent
1951–1952	18,700	7,900	42			
1952–1953	17,000	7,500	44			
1953–1954	17,800	7,700	43			
1954–1955	18,900	8,300	44			
1955–1956	19,000	7,300	39			
1956–1957	20,300	9,600	47			
1957–1958	19,800	8,100	40			
1958–1959	19,900	7,300	37	3,800	1,600	45
1959–1960	19,800	7,500	38	4,000	2,000	50
1960–1961	19,000	7,500	40	4,100	1,700	41
1961–1962	19,800	6,900	35	4,300	1,600	37
1962–1963	20,600	6,700	32	5,600	1,700	30
1963–1964	18,300	6,800	37	5,600	1,900	34
1964–1965	19,600	7,700	39	6,800	2,000	30
1965–1966	19,900	6,200	31	8,400	2,400	29
1966–1967	19,500	7,000	36	10,200	3,100	30
1967–1968	18,400	6,900	38	11,400	3,900	30

N.B.   (i) Figures taken to nearest hundred.

(ii) The numbers of students entered are those shown in the annual reports of the Council as "admitted for the first time".

(iii) Those discontinued are as shown in the report as "withdrawn on discontinuing training less number readmitted having previously discontinued training".

(iv) The figures are not strictly comparable but over a period of years show the trend.

(v) 1901—Wastage in Poor Law Institutions, 33 per cent approximately.

1930—Wastage in Local Authority and Voluntary Hospitals (complete training Schools)—26–28 per cent.[1]

Reference

1. A History of the Nursing Profession, p. 151. Abel Smith.

Appendix 5(iv)

NUMBER OF HOSPITALS APPROVED AS TRAINING SCHOOLS FOR ALL PARTS OF THE REGISTER

		Sick Children's	Fever	Mental	Mental Subnormality
At November 1949	878				
At March 1951	941				
1951–1952	989				
1952–1953	990				
1953–1954	984				
1954–1955	657 incl. 357 complete training schools within one hospital	25	60	125	48
1955–1956	658 ,, 357	25	54	125	48
1956–1957	643 ,, 349	25	38	127	49
1957–1958	624 ,, 296	25	34	127	48
1958–1959	611 ,, 293	25	33	126	49
1959–1960	600 ,, 289	25	29	126	51
1960–1961	590 ,, 280	24	23	126	51
1961–1962	580 ,, 272	24	23	127	51
1962–1963	564 ,, 267	24	21	127	52
1963–1964	467 ,, 100	23	17	126	57
1964–1965	456 ,, 95	23	14	126	57
1965–1966	428 ,, 95	22	12	127	57
1966–1967	425 ,, 96	22	—	121	57

N.B. (i) These figures are as shown in the annual reports of the General Nursing Council.
(ii) The 1967/1968 figures are not given since, due to the grouping of many training schools, the "Council's analysis has been presented in a different form and details cannot be compared with those shown in previous annual reports."

Appendix 5(*v*)

NUMBER OF HOSPITALS APPROVED AS
TRAINING SCHOOLS FOR THE ROLL OF NURSES

At November 1949	128
At March 31st, 1951	210
1951–1952	285
1952–1953	335
1953–1954	371
1954–1955	400
1955–1956	426
1956–1957	459
1957–1958	479
1958–1959	513
1959–1960	515
1960–1961	526
1961–1962	552
1962–1963	586
1963–1964	625
1964–1965	641
1965–1966	785

(including 138 Mental and Mental Subnormality Hospitals)

1966–1967	903

(including 182 Mental and Mental Subnormality Hospitals)

1967/1968 figures not given. See note (ii) Appendix 5(iv).

Appendix 5(vi)

EXPERIMENTAL SCHEMES OF TRAINING APPROVED BY COUNCIL

	4 Year S.R.N./R.S.C.N.	4 Year S.R.N./R.M.N.	18/12 or 15/12 second training	S.R.N./R.F.N.	Special	No. of students
1951–1952	3		1 Psychiatric	4		—
1952–1953	8		4	4		164 involved
1953–1954	9	1	13 "	7		127 indexed
1954–1955	9	4	24 "	10	1	583 "
1955–1956	10	9	44 "	6	2	348 "
1956–1957	13	9	77 "	13	2	438 "
1957–1958	8	8	109 " and Sick Children	13	2	530 "
1958–1959	8	9	125 "	11	4	557 "
1959–1960	8	10	140 "	11	4	713 "
1960–1961	9	9	167 "	13	3	744 "
1961–1962	9	9	207 "	13	3	827 "
1962–1963	10	9	257 "	12	6	1,111 "
1963–1964	9	8	318 "	4	6	1,210 "
1964–1965	10	9	49 "	4	7	1,443 "
1965–1966	10	9	57 "	—	9	1,200 "
1966–1967	10	8	71 "	—	12	893 "
1967–1968	11	8	72 "	—	21	859 "

N.B.—18/12 Schemes of training ceased to be experimental in 1964.

Appendix 6

ELECTIONS 1923–1965

	Seats	Nominations	Electorate		Per cent vote	
1923	16	31	Over	12,000	approx.	66
1927	16	27	,,	50,000	,,	44
1932	16	32	,,	62,000	,,	35
1937	16	50	,,	86,000	,,	41
1944	16	37	,,	119,000	,,	36
1950	17	151	,,	145,000	,,	31
1955	17	69	,,	183,000	,,	31
1960	17	66	,,	217,000	,,	25
1965	18	43	,,	266,000	,,	25

N.B. (i) 1949 Act: Changed the constitution of the General Nursing Council (16–17 seats)
Retention Fee abolished
Consolidated Registration Fee introduced.

(ii) 1965 Election: 1 new seat—Wessex Region.

(iii) Electorate: Since 1950 when the Consolidated Fee was introduced the electorate figure given above is the number of voting papers known to have been delivered.

INDEX OF SUBJECTS

INDEX OF NAMES